Herbal Primer

Cara E. Moore, BSYA (Crys.)(Herb.)

(FMANF) Yoga Teaching (Hatha Yoga)

DEDICATION

I would like to dedicate this book to the British School of Yoga for their practitioner training in Herbalism and Making Aromatherapy and Natural Health Product courses. Also to my son Christopher who shares my love of herblore and got me the mortar and pestle set shown on the cover to celebrate my graduation.

CONTENTS

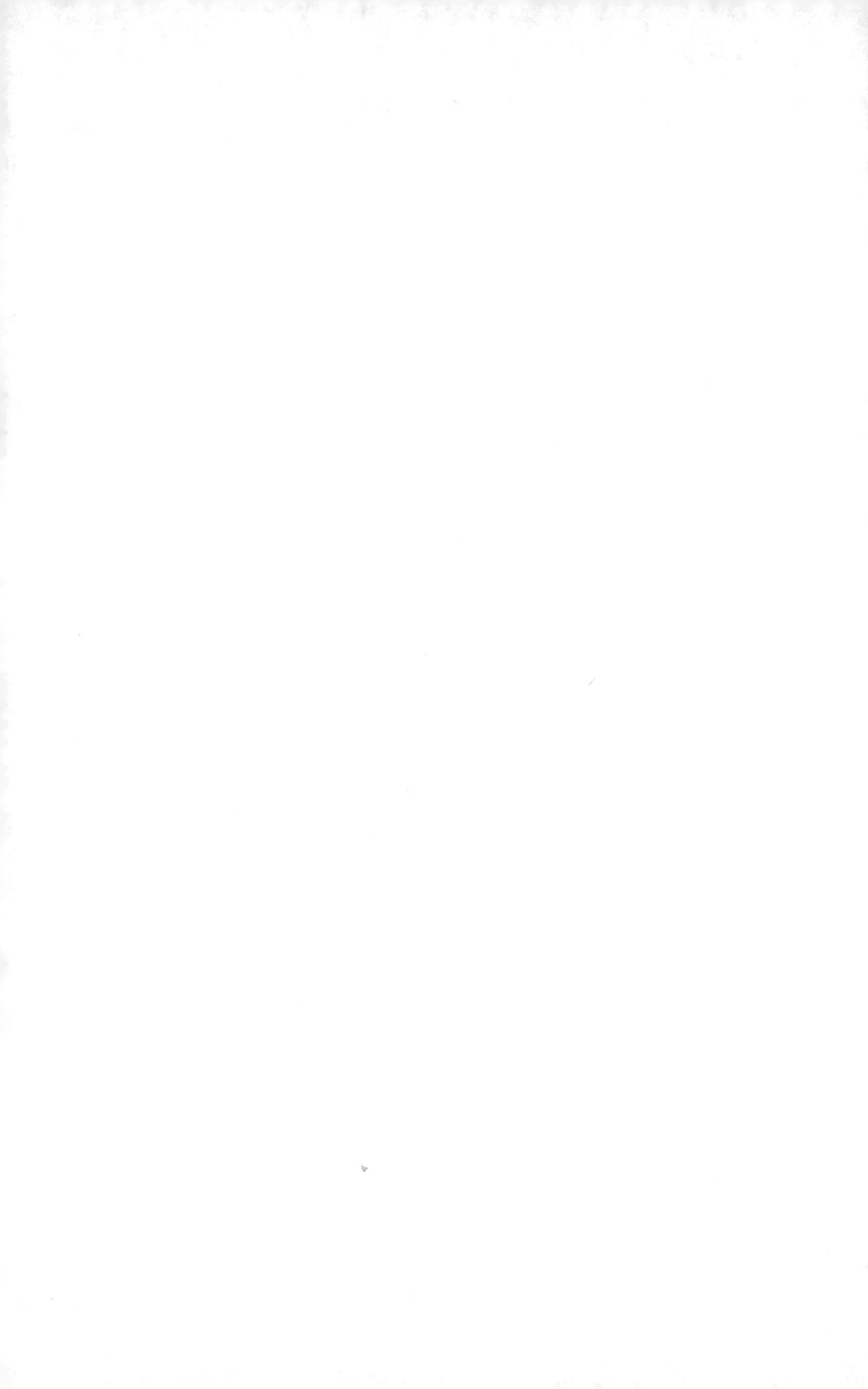

ACKNOWLEDGMENTS

I would like to acknowledge the British School of Yoga for their training and my herbal suppliers for their products and information and the organizations dedicated to promoting herbal knowledge such as Baldwins, The Herb Society, the Royal Horticultural Society and the American Botanical Council.

1 HISTORY OF HERBAL HEALING

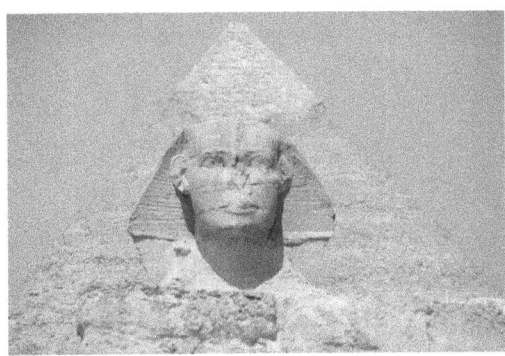

Sphinx, Egypt

Ancient Egyptians used hundreds of herbs for healing and rituals. The *Ebers Papyrus* dates from around 3550 BC. Ancient writing of Hippocrates (lived 460 to 370 BC) and *Materia Medica* (Science of Healing Drugs) of Pelanius Dioscurides (AD 40 to 90) wrote a compendium of more than 500 plants that remained an authoritative reference into the 17th century.

Ayurvedic (Indian) herbal medicine has the *Sushruta Samhita* (Sushruta in the 6th century BC) describes 700 medicinal plants, 64 preparations from mineral sources, and 57 preparations based on animal sources.

TCM, Traditional Chinese Medicine also has a long history of herblore and practical applications. The *Shennong Bencao Jing,* compiled during the Han

Dynasty but dating back to a much earlier date, possibly 2700 B.C., lists 365 medicinal plants and their uses.

Medical schools known as Bimaristan began to appear from the 9th century in the medieval Islamic world, and Ibn al-Baitar described more than 1,400 different plants, foods and drugs, with over 300 of which were his own original discoveries, in the 13th century.

The nun Hildegard of Bingen (1098 – 1179) was an authority on medieval herbal medicine and wrote *Physica of Plants*.

The experimental scientific method was introduced into the field of Materia Medica in the 13th century by the Andalusian an Arab botanist Abu al-Abbas al-Nabati, the teacher of Ibn al-Baitar. Al-Nabati introduced empirical techniques in the testing, description and identification of numerous Materia Medica, and he separated unverified reports from those supported by actual tests and observations.

Both Henry the Eighth and Elizabeth the First were avid herbalist, Henry the Eighth passed laws (1543) allowing people to continue to practice Herbal medicine so the ordinary person would have access to medical care.

The English Physician Enlarged (1653) by Nicholas Culpeper included traditional medicine with astrology, magic, and folklore was ridiculed by the physicians of his day yet was very popular. *The Age of Exploration* and the *Columbian Exchange* introduced new medicinal plants to Europe. *The Badianus Manuscript* was an illustrated Aztec herbal translated into Latin in the 16th century.

The WHO recognizes that for most of the world, herbal treatments are used as a necessity and Herblore is a vital tradition.

Further herbal resources

http://www.herbalremediesinfo.com/best-herbal-remedies.html

http://www.baldwins.co.uk

http://www.herbsociety.org.uk

http://www.rhs.org.uk/

http://abc.herbalgram.org/site/PageServer

2 HERBALISM

Herbalism is a healing art that sees the person in a holistic manner, the mind, the body, the spirit, as one. Lifting one's frame of mind with Aromatherapy or an herbal tea is as important as making a poultice for a boil or rash. It is about bringing balance back in a gentle, nurturing way that limits side-effects.

When visiting an Herbalist a history of the patient is taken. The goals of the treatment are discussed, be it Stress, troubling sleeping, general run-down feeling or something more specific such as a rash or Anxiety. It is important to complete this history, to ensure no detrimental interaction occurs between prescription drugs and conditions and herbal treatments. There are fewer side effects with herbal treatments because the concentration of dosage is lower, but all herbs have to be used with a healthy respect.

Teas and herbal baths are the most gentle introduction and if they prove effective, capsules can be made for more ease of convenience. (such as ground Feverfew for a migraine).

Aromatherapy is an important part of Herbalism. Essential oils are extremely concentrated and must be mixed with carrier oils and reduced to ¼ of the dose for infants over 1 month old, such as chamomile or lavender. It is not recommended to use more stimulating essential oils as it puts a strain on a young child's metabolism.

Most herbal teas and treatments used should show a result within 3 days and should be discontinued immediately if any adverse reaction occurs.

Herbalism is seen as a complementary medicine and an Herbalist will refer a client to a doctor for clarification of symptoms. One of the major benefits of Herbal treatment is its individual nature. Different combination of herbs are used to facilitate this nature of approach. Sometimes when a person is very unwell; a combination of conditions are present, herbs are used to bring the body back into balance, boosting the body's own healing process.

Diet and Exercise are also an important aspect of Herbal treatment. Meditation can also be used to calm the mind and body.

After the initial session, future sessions are used for feedback on the effects of treatment and any modifications needed are discussed and implemented.

Knowledge obtained for Herbalism is an ongoing process, such as recent study on Rosehips by the Frederiksberg Hospital in Copenhagen, Denmark . "Experts now believe the same rosehip ingredient may combat Rheumatoid Arthritis, Crohn's disease and even heart disease. All are conditions in which inflammation plays an important role. Biochemist Dr Kaj Winther, from Frederiksberg Hospital in Copenhagen, Denmark, who has a special interest in rosehips, said: "There's emerging evidence that the anti-inflammatory and antioxidant compounds in rosehips might have quite a wide therapeutic effect." A small trial run by Dr. Winther showed that an herbal remedy made from the ground up seeds and shells of hips from the dog rose, Rosa canina, had a big impact on the pain of osteoarthritis.

More than 80% of the 94 Danish men and women with arthritic hips, knees or hands who took part in the study on rosehips reported a significant reduction in pain after taking the supplement for three weeks. They also cut their consumption of standard painkillers by 50%. The findings, published in the Scandinavian

Journal of Rheumatology last year, followed a Norwegian study which found that restricted movement caused by osteoarthritis was reduced by 40% in patients taking rosehips. Herbal preparation, with the exception of essential oils, which is a complicated process, is within reach of most people, tinctures, poultices, infused oils, herbal teas and powders into capsules can all be done by hand.

3 AROMATHERAPY USES

Aromatherapy uses the healing power of essential oils to heal the mind and body.

Aniseed: Latin: Pimpinella anisum (extracted from seed of plant) Herbal Classifications: Anti-spasmodic, (useful for period pains) carminative, helpful for asthma, colds, sore throats. Galactagogue, helps stimulate milk flow. Anti-parasitic, useful to treat lice and scabies. Caution: Irritant to sensitive skin, stimulant.

Basil: Latin: Ocimum basilicum Herbal Classification: Nerve tonic, aids concentration. Caution: Stimulant

Benzion: Latin: Styrax benzion Herbal Action Classification: Vanilla like aroma, helps circulation, inhalation, laryngitis, upper respiratory conditions, warming

Bergamot: Latin: Citrus aurantium sub bergamia (from fruit peel) Herbal Classifications: Anti-depressant, Relaxant, Antiseptic, acne, ulcers, Chicken pox, shingles, cold sores, wounds, inhalation for lung conditions. Relaxant. Caution: Phototoxic, do not use before exposure to sun. Used to flavor Earl Grey Tea

Black Pepper: Latin: Piper Nigrum (Black Pepper) Seed Oil Herbal Action Classifications: Used for muscular aches, bad circulation, use in bath to stop "flu" conditions. Caution: Stimulant.

Camphor: Herbal Action Classifications: First aid remedy as a cold compress bruises, sprain, reduces swelling Caution: Strong stimulant, don't take internally.

Caraway: Latin: Carum carvi (from seed of plant) Herbal Action Classifications: Folklore believed would prevent a theft. Carminative, digestive complaints, Galactagogue, (useful for breast feeding) Caution: May cause dermal irritation.

Cedarwood: Latin: Juniperus virginiana Herbal Action Classifications: Inhalant respiratory infections with excess catarrh, dandruff, arthritis, rheumatism. Caution: Do not take internally, not for use during pregnancy, irritant to sensitive skins.

Chamomile: Latin: Anthemis Nobilis (from flower of plant) Herbal Action Classifications: Soothing for calm & Anxiety. For insomnia use in late bath, relaxes muscles. Cooling febrifuge, carminative, speeds us wound healing, prevents gastric ulcers. Inhalations help relieve bacterial toxins. Anti-inflammatory. Caution: Can be an irritation for those with sensitive skins.

Cinnamon: Latin: Cinnamomum zeylanicum (bark) Herbal Action Classifications: Exhaustion, after flu, helps digestion, stimulate the heart, strong antiseptic, inhalation. Caution: Irritant to sensitive skin Promotes appetite, Carminative

Citronella: Latin: Cymbopogon nardus (grass) Herbal Action Classifications: Rheumatic pain (Chinese use) diluted on temples for sleeplessness, insect repellent, neuralgia, migraine

Clary Sage: Latin: (Salvia Sclarea) (Flower tops) Herbal Action Classifications: Relaxing oil, helps insomnia Anti-inflammatory, relieves sore throats, hoarseness, inhalations, reduces high blood pressure, antispasmodic, relieves pmt, menstrual pain, soothes swollen breasts, helps prevent hot flushes Caution: Relaxant. May cause sleepiness. Useful for Depression, anxiety, tension, mental fatigue, general tonic. Avoid during first five months of pregnancy.

Clove: Latin: Eugenia caryophyllus (dried flower buds) Herbal Action Classifications: Antiseptic, used as an inhalation or on the skin, treating tooth infections, pain. Helps lift mental and physical conditions. Caution: Skin irritant. Strong Antiseptic Anti-spasmodic (useful Asthma, Bronchitis) Prolonged use can damage gum tissues.

Cypress: Latin Cupressus sempervirens (twigs, needles and cones) Herbal Action Classifications: Good for flu, coughs, inhalation, clears sinuses, good massage oil for varicose veins, helps menstrual problems. Can help staunch hemorrhage, useful after childbirth as a means of controlling blood lost, calming vulval tissue. Cautions: Useful for Cramps, Rheumatism. Avoid if you have high blood pressure.

Eucalyptus: Latin: Eucalyptus globules (fresh leaves of tree) Herbal Action Classifications: Strong, anti-microbial oil, inhalation, direct skin application for chicken pox, cold sores, shingles, insect repellent. Diuretic, muscular sprain, rheumatoid arthritis, applied as rub for respiratory infections. Caution: Very strong, use sparingly. Useful as air spray in sick rooms. Useful in bringing high temperatures down (cold compress) monitor carefully to prevent shock.

Sweet Fennel: Latin: Foeniculum vulgate (seed of plant) Herbal Action Classifications: Carminative, laxative, eases wind, hiccoughs, indigestion, colic, massage oil for cellulitis. Galactagogue, (improves milk flow) useful for menopause. Folklore, used to prevent evil eye, hung over doorway. Caution: Phototoxic, not to be used on sensitive sking. Useful for Gout, alcohol poisoning. Expectorant, useful in massage rubs on abdomen, Lower back massage for flatulence and constipation. Tea useful for diarrhea, colic, appetite stimulant.

Frankincense: Latin: Boswellia thurifear (bark) Herbal Action Classifications: Eases anxiety, good inhalation for respiratory problems. Astringent, uterine tonic, for heavy periods, labour, after birth, cystitis, helps heal stubborn wounds heal. Caution: Useful for Asthma, calms.

Ginger: Latin: Zingiber Officinale Herbal Action Classifications: Rubefacient for rheumatic aches and pains. Good general tonic, used in bath to help prevent infections and colds. Caution: Stimulant.

Hyssop: Latin: Hyssopus officinalis Herbal Action Classifications: General nerve tonic, helps regulate blood pressure either high or low. Caution:

Sedative

Jasmine: Latin: Jasminum Officinale Herbal Action Classifications: Anti-depressent, aphrodisiac, eases pain of whole female reproduction system.

Juniper: Latin: Juniperus communic (dried berries) Herbal Action Classifications: Appetite stimulant, urinary tract, skin, gout, respiratory, detoxifier, piles (diluted) weeping eczema, dermatitis, acne. Caution: Avoid if pregnant, severe kidney disease.

Lavender: Latin: Lavandula officinalis (fresh flowers) Herbal Action Classifications: Eases aches & pains, useful for migraines and headaches. Cytophylactc, stimulates cell growth, relieves spasms, period pains (hot compress of lavender) Sinusitis, catarrhal coughs, sore throats, congestion, general tonic during and after illness. Caution: Relaxant. Treatment of burns, anti-spasmodic, analgesic, lessens scarring, cold compress forehead, back of neck for headaches, migraines, stress, shock, worry, impatience.

Lemon: Latin: Citrus Medica Limonum (Lemon) Peel Oil Herbal Action Classifications: Good remedy for sore throats, gargle with 2% oil to warm water, antiseptic use on insect bites and stings, use straight on warts and verrucas.

Lemongrass: Latin: Cymbopogon citrates (grass) Herbal Classifications: stimulating oil, cleanses oily skin. Antibacterial, anti-fungal, useful for infections, feverish conditions, used in Indian medicine. Cautions: General tonic, strong odour, protects animals from ticks, fleas, colitis, muscular aches, pains.

Marigold: Latin: Calendula officinalis Herbal Classifications: Vulnerary (healing oil). Reduces inflammation, helps chilblains, chapped or cracked skin, excellent for bruises and burns.

Marjoram: Latin: Origanum majorana Herbal Classifications: useful for anxiety, grief, insomnia, eases muscular, menstrual and rheumatic, helps migraines. Caution: Warming: Avoid during first five months of pregnancy. Useful for Asthma, lowers high blood pressure, colic.

Myrrh: Latin Commiphora myrrha Herbal Classifications: strong healer, antiseptic, anti-catarrhal, inhalation will help most respiratory conditions.

Neroli: Latin: Citrus aurantium (flowers from tree) Herbal Classifications: stress, colitis, palpitations, insomnia, diarrhea, scarring, thread veins, stretch marks, dry, sensitive skin.

Orange Flower: Latin: Citrus Aurantium Dulcis (Orange) Peel Oil Herbal Classifications: Anxiety, palpitations, eases depression, shock and fear.

Parsley: Latin Petroselinum crispum (seeds) Herbal Classifications: emmenagogue, Diuretic, Febrifuge (brings down temperature) Digestion, tonic effect on uterus, used during labour. Caution: Do not use in pregnancy. Useful for asthma, circulator tonic, used in piles ointment (Anti-inflammatory)

Peppermint: Latin Mentha piperita Herbal Classifications: Digestion, nausea, irritable bowel syndrome, eases migraine, insect repellent. Relieves mastitis, fever. Shock, hysteria, paralysis, palpitation from shock, Dysmenorrhoea, anti-rheumatic. Caution: Do not use when pregnant, irritant to sensitive skin. Antiseptic. Eye irritant. alleviates headaches, cold compress or inhalation, travel sickness. In massage oil for indigestion, stomach pains, flatulence, irritable bowel syndrome.

Pine: Latin: Pinus sylvestris (needles, twigs, cones) Herbal Classifications: Antiseptic Oil, helps clears mind, eases mental fatigue. Strong antiseptic, expectorant, decongestant, circulation stimulant, respiratory conditions, bronchitis, sinusitis. Sore throat, flu, pneumonia. Caution: Make sure is Pinus sylvestirs. Other species may be hazardous. Gout, muscular pains, arthritis, rheumatism, neuralgia, nervous diseases.

Rose: Latin: Rosa damascena Herbal Classifications: Soothing to nerves, anti-depressant, calms anger, eases hangovers.

Rose Geranium: Latin: Pelargonium graveolens (leaves and flowers from plant) Herbal Classification: Insect repellent. Antiseptic, haemostatic (helps stop bleeding) regulates hormonal imbalances, PMT, cellulites and mastitis, diarrhea, peptic ulcers, eczema, burns, shingles, ringworm, lice, anti-fungal. Caution: Irritant to sensitive skins. Useful for anxiety.

Rosemary: Latin: Rosmarinus officinalis (leaves of plant) Herbal Classifications: Stimulates weak memory, eases dullness and headaches. Helps prevents muscle strain, emmenagogue, anti-bacterial, anti-oxidant, sciatica. Poor circulation, varicose veins, arthritis, inhalation for respiratory illnesses, digestive, flatulence, stomach pains, constipation, dandruff, astringent tonic for oily skin. Caution: avoid during pregnancy. Stimulant. Adds shine to dark hair when used as a rinse. Not to be used before bed, as stimulates. Do not use if you have high blood pressure.

Sage: Latin: Salvia officinalis (whole herb) Helps prevent sweating, anti-inflammatory, Period Pains, Menopausal, sore throats, Oral Thrush, Gingivitis, Laryngitis. Caution: Not to be swallowed when used in mouth gargle.

Sandalwood: Latin: Santalum album (drips, rasping of heart wood of tree) Herbal Action Classification: Anxiety, nervous tension. Diuretic, Anti-spasmodic, respiratory infections, expectorant, can be applied to throat, massage into chest and back, soothing action on dry, sore or inflamed skin

Tea Tree: Latin: Melaleuca alternifolia (leaves of plant) Herbal Action Classification: Antiseptic, anti-viral, anti-fungal, anti-bacterial, antiseptic, thrush, cystitis, respiratory infections, cold sores, lice. Cautions: Acne, burns, sunburn, (in a cream)

Thyme: Latin Thymus vulgaris (flowers of plant) Herbal Action Classification: Powerful antiseptic. Digestion, expectorant, emmenagogue, diuretic, anti-spasmodic, carminative, respiratory, colds, convulsive coughing, whooping cough, asthma, mouth, throat, chest infection, stimulates appetite, depression in aftermath of illness. Stimulates immune system. Caution: Do not use neat on skin or during pregnancy, do not use on children's skin. Useful for gout, arthritis, muscles aches and sprains, boils, sores, infected skin conditions, insomnia, nervous anxiety, exhaustion.

Verbena: Latin: Verbena officinalis. Herbal Action Classification: Nerve tonic, eases and strengthens, anxiety, palpitations, dizziness, insect repellent

Ylang-Ylang: Latin: Cananga odorata (flowers) Aphrodisiac, sense of well-being, anxiety, tension, anger. Tachycardia, palpitations, hyperpnoea, high blood pressure.

4 HERBAL ACTION CLASSIFICATIONS

Adaptogen

Herbs that enable the body to avoid reaching a point of collapse or overstress, Traditional Chinese Medicine, Ayurvedic concept. Example: Gingseng (Panax ginseng)

Alternative

Herbs that gradually restore the proper function of the body and increase health and vitality. Example: Burdock (Arctium lappa)

Anthelmintic

Herb that destroys or expels intestinal parasitic worms. Example: Garlic, (*Allium sativum*) Wormwood. (*Artemisia absinthum*)

Anti-bilious

Herbs that help the body to remove excess bile.   Example: Golden Seal (*Hydrastis canadenis*)

Anti-catarrhal

Herbs that help the body to remove excess catarrhal build-ups. Example: Elder (*Sambucus nigra*)

Anti-Depressive

Herbs similar in use to Thymoleptic, such as Nervine tonics.

Anti-emetic

Herbs that reduce nausea and can help to prevent vomiting. Example; Black Horehound (*Ballota nigra*)

Anti-haemorrhagic

Herbs that are astringent.

Anti-Inflamatory

Herbs that help the body to combat inflammations. Example Chamomile (*Matricaria chamomilla*)

Anti-lithic

Herbs that help prevent the formation of stones or gravel in the urinary system and help remove those already formed. Example: Parsley Piert (*Aphanes arvensis*)

Anti-Microbial

Herbs hat help the body to destroy or resist pathogenic microorganisms. Example: Echinacea (*Echinacea angustifilia*)

Anti-parasitic

Often used as a synonym for Anthelmintic.

Anti-pyretic

A synonym for Febrifuge.

Anti-spasmodic

Herbs that can prevent or ease spasms or cramps in the **muscles of the** body. Example: Crampbark (*Viburnum opulus*)

Aperient

Herb that is a mild and gentle form of laxative. Example: Rhubarb Root (*Rheum palmatum*)

Aromatic

An herb that has a distinctive pleasant smell. The oils are the basis of aromatherapy. Example: Aniseed (*Pimpinella anisum*)

Astringent

Herbs that that draws tissue together. Example: Agrimony (*Agrimonia eupatoria*)

Bitter

Herbs that help the detoxification of the liver, regulate blood sugar, repair gut wall damage, stimulate appetite, help allergy distorted digestion. Example: Gentian Root (*Gentiana lutea*)

Cardiac tonic

Herbs that have a beneficial action on the heart. Example: Lilly of the Valley (*Convallaia majalis*)

Carminative

Herbs that relieve flatulence or colic by expelling gas. Example: Fennel (*Foeniculum vulgare*)

Cholagogue

Herbs that stimulate the flow of bile from the liver. Example: Balmony (*Chelone glabra*)

Demulcent

Herbs that are rich in mucilage and can soothe and protect irritated or inflamed internal tissues. Example: Comfrey (*Symphytum officinale*)

Depurative

Same term as Alternative.

Diaphoretic

Herbs that induce sweating and help poor circulation. Example: Yarrow (*Achillea millefolium*)

Digestive Bitter

Same term as bitter.

Diurectic

Herbs that cause an increase of urine and help the body eliminate waste and support inner cleansing. Example: Bearberry (*Arctostaphylos uva-ursi*)

Emetic

Herbs that cause a person to vomit. Example: Ipecacuanha (*Cephaelis ipecacuanha*)

Emmenagogue

Herbs that stimulate menstral flow. Example: Blue Cohosh (*Caulophyllum thalictroides*)

Emollienta

Herbs that soften or soothes the skin. Example: Chickweed (*Stellaria media*)

Expectorant

A herb that stimulates the production of phlegm. Use: treatment of coughs. Example: Coltsfoot (*Tussilago farfara*)

Febrifuge

A herb that reduces fever. Example: Peppermint (*Mentha piperita*)

Galactagogue

Herbs that increase the production and secretion of milk. Example: Goat's Rue (*Galega officinalis*)

Hepatic

Herbs that tone, strengthen, and increase the flow of bile in liver. Example Dandelion (*Taraxacum officinale*)

Hypnotic

Herbs that help induce a deep and healing sleep. Example: Passionflower (*Passiflora incarnate*)

Laxative

Herbs that actively stimulate the bowels to promote movements. Example: Senna Pods (*Cassia angustifolia*).

Nervine

Herbs that have a beneficial effect upon the nervous system. Example: Oats (*Avena sativa*)

Pectoral

Herbs for chest or respiratory disorders. Example: Elecampane (*Inulahelenium*)

Rubefacient

A herb that causes the skin to become red as a counterirritant. Example: Mustard (*Brassica alba*)

Sedative

Herb that calms the nervous system and reduces stress and nervousness throughout the body. Example: Valerian (*Valeriana officinalis*)

Spasmolytic

An herb that controls muscle spasms. Same as antispasmodic.

Stimulant

Herb that quickens and enlivens the physiological activity of the body. Example: Bayberry (*Myrica cerifera*)

Styptic

A herb that slows down the rate of bleeding, same as astringent.

Thymoleptic

Herbs that raise the mood and counteracts depression. Example: Damiana (*Turnera aphrodisiaca*)

Tonic

Herbs that strengthen and enliven a specific organ or the whole body. Example: Golden Seal (*Hydrastis canadensis*)

Vulnerary

Herb used for treating and healing wounds. Example: Marigold (*Calendula officinalis*)

5 HERBS FOR THE BODY SYSTEM

Digestive System

A good balanced whole food diet is the foundation for good digestive health.

Demulcents: Comfrey root, Marshmallow root, Slippery elm

Meadowsweet (*Filipendula ulmaria*) It acts to protect and sooth digestive tract, reduces excess acidity and eases nausea. Used in treatment of heartburn, hyperactivity, gastritis and peptic ulceration. Useful in treating diarrhoea in children, reduces fever, eases pain of rheumatism in muscles and joints.

Dosage: Pour a cup of boiling water onto 1-2 tsp. of dried herb and leave to infuse for 10-15 minutes. Drink x 3 a day as needed.

Bitters: These remedies aid digestion. Gentian, Golden Seal, Rue, Milder bitters - Yarrow and Centaury.

Astringents: (useful for inflammatory, diarrhoeal states) Example: Bayberry and Yarrow

Constipation: Dandelion, Yellow Dock or Rhubarb root. Stronger herb would be Senna.

Anti-spasmodic : Colic pain: Chamomile and Peppermint, Hops.

The Mouth

Echinacea and Myrrh will help keep the mouth healthy. Mouth ulcers can be treated with Red Sage (*Salvia officinalis*). Traditional treatment of inflammation of mouth, throat and tonsils, soothes mucous membranes. Used internally and as a mouthwash for inflamed gums, as a gargle in the treatment of Laryngitis, Pharyngitis, Tonsillitis and Quinsy. **Caution: Avoid during pregnancy.** Dosage: Pour a cup of boiling water onto 1-2 tsp of the leaves and let infuse for 10 minutes, drink 3 times a day. Mouthwash, put 2 tsp of the leaves in half a litre of water, bring to the boil and let stand, covered for 15 minutes. Gargle deeply with the hot tea for 5 - 10 minutes several times a day.

Peptic ulcer

Marshmallow Root, Comfrey Root, Slippery Elm.

Irritable Bowel Syndrome

Chamomile, Hops, Wild Yam, Fennel, Peppermint.

Liver and Pancreas

Milder hepatics, cholagogues and bitters help and support the action of the liver. Dandelion root, Vervain, Balmony and Milk Thistle.

Cardio-Vascular System

Cardiac tonics: Lilly of the Valley, Hawthorn Berries, Broom, Motherwort, Bugleweed and Figwort.

Circulatory stimulants: Cayenne, Ginger, Prickly ash, Mustard, Rosemary and Horseradish. Dandelion for high potassium and diuresis, Broom and Yarrow as diuretics.

Heart Disease: Broom tops (*Sarothamnus scoparius*) increases the efficiency of each stroke of the heart, can be used where water retention occurs due to heart weakness and cases in over profuse menstruation. **Caution do not use Broom in pregnancy or hypertension.** Dosage: Pour a cup of boiling water onto 1 tsp of the dried herb and infuse for 10-15   minutes, drink x 3 a day.

Blood Pressure

Lime Blossom (*Tilia europea*) Has a reputation as a prophylactic against the development of arteriosclerosis and hypertension. Dosage: Pour a cup of boiling water onto 1 tsp of the blossoms and infuse for 10 minutes drink x 3 a day. For effect in fever, use 2-3 tsp. Wood betony will ease headaches due to high blood pressure. Garlic eaten raw daily will lower blood pressure.

Low blood pressure

Hyssops – balances both high and low blood pressure. Combine with cardiovascular tonic Hawthorn. Broom, Hawthorn Berries, Oats, Kola, Gentian and Wormwood.

Anaemia

Parsley, Nettles, Apricots and Pumpkin Seeds. Bitter herbs to aid the digestive process. Gentian, Condurango and Wormwood.

Bad circulation

Cayenne, Ginger, Prickly Ash and Hawthorn.

Varicose Veins

Hawthorn Berries, Horsechestnut and Buckwheat. For water build-up Yarrow and Dandelion Leaf.

Horsechestnut (*Aesculus hippocastanum*)

Increases the strength and tone of the blood vessels. Dosage pour a cup of boiling water onto 1 - 2 tsp of the dried fruit and leave to infuse for 10 to 15 minutes drink x 3 a day or used as a lotion.

Respiratory System

Expectorants: Coltsfoot, Mullein, White Horehound, Aniseed, Hyssop, Angelica, Sweet Violet, Elecampane and Bloodroot.

Sweet Violet (*Viola odorata*) Dosage: Pour a cup of boiling water onto 1 tsp of the herb and let infuse for 10-15 minutes drink x 3 a day.

Pectoral

Strengthens and tones the tissue of the lungs Elecampane, Mullein, Lobelia, Coltsfoot

Anti-microbials – Echinacea, Wild Indigo and Myrrh, Garlic and Thyme.

Anti-catarrhal – Golden Rod, Golden Seal, Elder Flowers, Hyssops.

Potters Herbal Remedy for Cough

Marshmallow Flowers, Mallow Flowers

Coltsfoot Flower, Sweet Violet Flowers

Mullein Flowers, Red Poppy Flowers.

Mixed in equal parts and infuse.

Asthma

Sundew (*Drosera rotundiflolia*)

Its relaxing effect upon involuntary muscles helps in relief of asthma. Dosage: Pour a cup of boiling water onto 1 tsp of the dried herb and leave to infuse for 10-15 minutes drink x 3 a day.

Ear, Nose And Throat

Colds and Flu: Elder Flower, Peppermint, Yarrow and Ginger

Ear infections: St. John's Wort Oil, warm oil of Mullein. (infuse oil with Mullein, then drain)

Hayfever: Ephedra, Golden Rod, Golden Seal and Eyebright

The Throat: Red Sage

The Eye: Eyebright (*Euphrasio officinalis*)

Helpful in acute and chronic inflammation, stinging and weeping eyes as well as oversensitivity to light. Dosage: Pour a cup of boiling water onto 1 tsp of dried herb and infuse for 5-10 minutes drink x 3 a day. Compress:

place a tsp of dried herb in half a litre of water and boil for 10 minutes, let cool slightly. Moisten a compress in the lukewarm liquid, wring out slightly and place over eyes.

Lymphatic System

Cleavers, Marigold. Poke Root, Echinacea, Golden Seal, Wild Indigo, Blue Flag and Garlic

Cleaver (*Galium aparine*)

Tonic for lymphatic system, used in swollen glands, tonsillitis, adenoids, dry varieties of Psoriasis, Cystitis, ulcers and tumours. Dosage: Pour a cup of boiling water onto 2-3 tsp of dried herb and leave to infuse for 10-15 minutes drink x 3 a day.

Urinary System

Parsley. **Do not use in pregnancy in medicinal dosage.** Pour 1-2 tsp of leaves and infuse for 5 -10 minutes in a closed container. Drink x 3 a day.

Horsetail (*Equisetum arvemse*) Astringent for whole genito-urinary system. Pour a cup of boiling water onto 2 tsp of the dried plant and let infuse for 15-20 minutes, drink x 3 a day. Also useful as a bath for rheumatic pain.

Anti-lithics helps body get rid of renal stones and gravel.

Stone Root (*Collinsonia canadensis*)

Can be used as a prophylaxis. Dosage: put 1-3 tsp of the dried root in a cup of water, bring to boil and simmer for 10-15 minutes. Drink x 3 a day.

Bladder infections

Yarrow drink as infusion 3 to 4 times a day.

Reproductive System

Tonics: Blue Cohosh, False Unicorn Root, Life Root and Squaw

Vine

Blue Cohosh – strengthens uterus Put one tsp of dried root in a cup of water, bring to boil, simmer for 10 minutes, drink x 3 times **a day**.

Hormonal Normalisers Chasteberry (*Vitex agnus-castus*) Tonic for reproductive organs. Pour a cup of boiling water onto 1 tsp of ripe berries and leave to infuse for 10-15 minutes. Drink x 3 a day.

Menstrual Cycle Cramp Bark – painful periods.

PMT: Valerian, Motherwort, for herbal long – term treatment Chasteberry. For diuretics, Dandelion Leaf and Yarrow

Pregnancy and Childbirth

Raspberry leaves (*Rubus idaeus*) Strengthens womb. Pour a cup of boiling water onto 2 tsp of the dried herb and let infuse 10-15 minutes. This may be drunk freely.

Morning Sickness: Peppermint, Black Horehound, Chamomile

Increase milk production Goat's Rye, Fennel, Fenugreek and Aniseed

Decrease milk production liberal amounts of Red Sage

Menopause Chasteberry, Blue Cohosh, Life Root, False Unicorn Root, Golden Seal, Ladies Mantel, St. John's Wort, Motherwort, Pasque Flower, Skullcap and Valerian

Male Reproductive System

Saw Palmetto, Damiana and Ginseng. Ginseng general hormonal and endocrine adaptogen.

Saw Palmetto Berries (*Serenoa serrulata*) Put ½ to 1 tsp of berries in a cup of water, bring to boil, simmer gently for 5 minutes drink x 3 a day. Also used in enlargement of prostate.

The Nervous System

Stress: Oats, Chamomile, Lime blossom,   Wood Betony, Balm,

Lavender, Skullcap

Depression: Damiana (*Turnera aphrodisiaca*)

Strengthens the nervous system. Dosage: Pour a cup of boiling water onto 1 tsp of the dried leaves and infuse for 10-15 minutes drink x 3 a day.

Bitters lift depression as a general tonic: Wormwood, Mugwort, Rue and Gentian. Adoptogens - Ginseng

Sleep Remedies: Lavender oil added to bath, Valerian tea, Hops, Lime blossom, Passion flower, Wild lettuce.

Sleep Potion: Equal parts Skullcap, Valerian and Passion flower.

Tension Headaches: Wood Betony (*Stachys betonica*) Dosage: Pour a cup of boiling water onto 1-2 tsp of dried herb and leave to infuse for 10-15 minutes drink x 3 a day.

Migraine

Feverfew (*Tanacetum parthenium*)

Do not use during pregnancy. Use equivalent of one fresh leave 1-3 times a day. Also relieves painful periods and sluggish menstrual flow.

Hyperactivity: Red Clover. Lime Blossom, Chamomile

Pain and Neuralgia: St. John's Wort for longstanding neuralgic pain, use externally as an oil for three weeks. Valerian, Wild Lettuce.

Musculo-Skeletal System

Guaiacum (*Guaiacum officinale*)

Rheumatic complaints, treatment of Gout. Dosage: Pour 1 tsp of the wood chip in a cup of water, bring to boil and simmer for 15-20 minutes.

Celery Seed (*Apium graveolens*) – Anti-rheumatic. **Devils Claw** (*Harpagophytum procumbens*)– inflammation of joints.

Sprains - Distilled Witch Hazel eases pain and swelling, Arnica (lotion, bath or compress) bath remedies, Ginger or Thyme.

The Skin

Burdock Root, Cleavers, Figwort (**Caution: should be avoided if irregular heart beat**) Golden Seal, Poke Root, Yellow Dock, Red Clover (childhood eczema)

Chickweed (*Stellaria media*)

Dosage: Pour a cup of boiling water onto 2 tsp of the dried herb and infuse 5 minutes. Drink x 3 a day. External use chickweed into an ointment, to ease itching, a strong infusion can be added to bath water.

Hair and Scalp

Chamomile – light hair

Rosemary good for dark hair

Rosemary (*Rosemarinus officinalis*) Externally used to ease muscular pains, sciatica, neuralgia. Dosage pour a cup of boiling water onto 1-2 tsp of dried herb, infuse in covered container for 10-15 minutes drink x 3 a day.

Allergies and Auto-immune problems

Elder Flower, and berry, Eyebright, Garlic, Golden Rod, Golden Seal, Nettles and Peppermint

Ephedra (*Ephedra sinica*) Dosage: Put 1-2 tsp of dried herb in one cup of water, bring to boil and simmer for 10—15 minutes drink x 3 a day. Used to treat asthma, bronchitis, whooping cough.

Endocrine Glands

Liquorice (*Glycyrrhiza glabra*) Put ½ to 1 tsp of the root in a cup of water, bring to boil and simmer for 10-15 minutes drink x 3 a day. Used in treatment of adrenal gland problems, such as Addison's disease. Use as a

Treatment for peptic ulceration, gastritis and ulcers, relief of abdominal colic, Bronchitis conditions.

Borage (*Borago officinalis*)

Used as a restorative agent on the adrenal cortex. Borage may be used as a tonic for adrenals over a period of time, used during fevers and convalescence. Used in conditions such as Pleurisy. Leaves and seeds stimulate milk in nursing mothers. Dosage: Pour a cup of boiling water onto 2 tsp of dried herb and leave to infuse for 10-15 minutes. Drink x 3 a day.

Thyroid Gland

Over-activity **Bugleweed** (*Lycopus europaeus*)

Tightness of breathing, palpitation that occurs of nervous origin, aids weak heart and as a sedative cough reliever to ease irritating coughs of nervous origin. Dosage: Pour a cup of boiling water onto 1 tsp of dried herb and infuse for 10-15 minutes drink x 3 a day.

Bladderwrack (*Fucus vesiculosus*)

Used in treatment of underactive thyroid glands and goitre. Helps in reducing excess weight.

Relieves rheumatism and rheumatoid arthritis, both internally and external application upon inflamed joints. Pour a cup of boiling water onto 2-3 tsp dried herb, leave steep for 10 minutes drink x 3 a day.

Pancreas: Goat's Rue and bitters helps to kick start the glands.

Fevers and Infection

Diaphoretics: Promote sweating. Boneset, Yarrow, Vervain, Elder Flower, Hyssop, Lime Flower, Peppermint, Rosemary, Ginger and Cayenne

Circulatory Stimulates: Ginger, Cayenne, Mustard, Horseradish, Prickly Ash

Anti-microbials: Echinacea, Wild Indigo, Garlic, Myrrh

Diuretics: Aid and support kidney function

Nervines: Helpful in dealing with post infection depression or with extremes of delirium during a fever – Vervain.

Infections Ear Nose And Throat: Garlic, Echinacea, Wild Indigo, Golden Seal, Eucalyptus, Thyme, Balm of Gilead

The Lungs: Garlic, Echinacea, Elecampane, Blood Root, White Horehound, Aniseed Oil, Eucalyptus oil and Coltsfoot

Digestive: Garlic, Meadowsweet and Golden Seal. Worms - Wormwood, Tansy, Garlic Rue and Southernwood

Urinary: Bearberry, Juniper, Yarrow, Couch Grass, Buchu and Echinacea

Reproductive System: Echinacea, Wild Indigo, Nasturtium, Blue Cohosh

Musculoskeletal system: Black Willow, Bogbean and Devil's Claw

Nerves: St. John's Wort, Echinacea, Pasque Flower and Peppermint Oil

Skin Infection: Pasque Flower, Garlic, Echinacea, Eucalyptus Oil and Myrrh

6 HERBAL IDENTIFICATION

Caution: If you are taking any other medication, check to see if there will be an interaction with the listed herbs, website http://www.baldwins.co.uk/perl/go.pl/healthnotes.html?%2fuk%2fassets%2fa-z-index%2fa-to-z-index-of-vitamin-and-herb-interactions%2f%7edefault

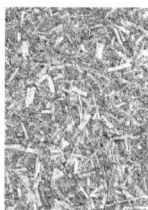

Agrimony *(Agrimonia eupatoria)*

Astringent, tonic, diuretic, vulnerary, cholagogue. A bitter tonic of the digestive system and liver, used in treatment of diarrhoea for children and mucous colitis. Traditional used as a "Spring Tonic" to wake up the digestive system. Used for urinary incontinence and cystitis. As a gargle for sore throats, Laryngitis, ointment for healing wounds and bruises. Dosage: Pour a cup of boiling water onto 1-2 tsp of the dried herb and infuse 10-15 minutes, drink x 3 a day.

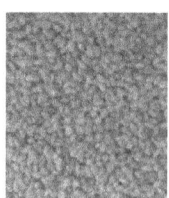

Alfalfa Seed
Alfalfa is rich in many nutrients hich includes calcium, potassium, iron and vitamins C, D, E and K. Restores strength to the sick and weak. Used to treat digestive weaknesses. Alfalfa seed sprouts have cooling properties used for disorders related to heat and inflammation. Used for treatment

for cystitis, lowering fevers and lowering cholesterol, diabetes, ulcers, arthritis and rheumatic problems and lower back ache.

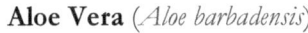

Alkanet Root *(Alkana tinctoria)*

Root used as a dye. Recipe for lip gloss: from Herbmoonhollow

Luscious Lips

2tsp alkanet root, 8oz almond or Grapeseed oil 2oz beeswax 1 tbsp honey Orange essential oil. Simmer alkanet in oil for about 15-20 minutes, or until the oil has turned a deep red/black colour. The deeper the colour the redder the oil will be when strained and bottled. Strain, add beeswax, honey & essential oil.

Aloe Vera *(Aloe barbadensis)*

Aloe vera extracts have antibacterial and antifungal properties, used as a moisturizer and for burn treatment. Internal intake of Aloe vera has been linked with improved blood glucose levels in diabetics, and with lower blood lipids in hyperlipidaemic patients and those with acute hepatitis (liver disease). Oral Aloe vera gel may reduce symptoms and inflammation in patients with ulcerative colitis. Used topically and internally for treatment of skin conditions such as eczema.

Angelica *(Angelica archangelica)*

Carminative, anti-spasmodic, expectorant, diuretic, diaphoretic. Expectorant for coughs, bronchitis and pleurisy, especially with fever, colds or influenza, used as a compress in inflammations of the chest, carminative for intestinal colic and flatulence, digestive stimulate used in treatment of anorexia nervosa, rheumatic inflammations, for cystitis as urinary antiseptic. Dosage: 1 tsp cut root in a cup of water, bring to boil and simmer for two minutes, let stand 15 minutes, take one cup x 3 a day.

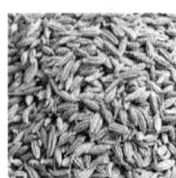

Aniseed (*Pimpinella anisum*)Expectorant, anti-spasmodic, carminative, parasiticide, aromatic intestinal colic, and flatulence, expectorant and anti-spasmodic used in bronchitis with irritable coughing, whooping cough, externally oil is used in treatment of scabies and to control and eradicate lice, used for flavouring. Dosage: Pour one cup of boiling water over 1-2 tsp of seeds, let stand covered for 5 -10 minutes, take one cup x 3 a day, tea should be drunk slowly before meals to prevent flatulence. If taking oil one drop oil taken internally by mixing with half a teaspoon of honey.

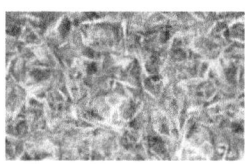

Arnica *(Arnica Montana)* Been used for centuries for oedema (fluid retention) and swelling, bruises, cuts, arthritis, sore muscles and joints, sore throats, swollen insect bites, and phlebitis. Has been approved by the European Commission for fever and colds, inflammation of the skin, cough/bronchitis, inflammation of the mouth and Pharynx, Rheumatism, common cold, blunt injuries and to prevent infection. **Caution: Do not take internally or put on open wounds.**

Ashwagandha Root Powder (*Withania somnifera*) Indian Adaptogen herb (similar properties to that of Ginseng) used to alleviate symptoms associated with arthritis. Reported to have anti-carcinogenic effects.

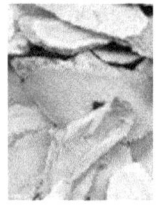

Astragulas Root (*Astragalus membranaceus*) General tonic and specifically for boosting the immune system. Used in TCM. Treats colds and flu, Angina, Hepatitis, Kidney & bladder infections, Alzheimer's disease, Chemotherapy support, Anti-tumour. Digestion, IBS. Dosage: Simmer 6 slices in 3 cups of water 1 hour. Strain and serve.

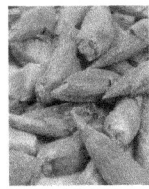

Balm of Gilead (*Poplar Buds*) – (*Populus candicans*), Anti-inflammatory, Antimicrobial, Analgesic. Used to treat sore throats, urinary problems. Traditionally soaked in olive oil and used as a balm.

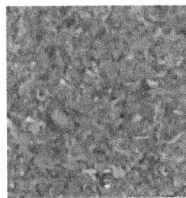

Basil (*Ocimum basilicum*) Used to treat stomach cramps, sickness, fevers, colds, flu, headaches and menstrual pain. Dosage: Pour a cup of boiling water onto 1-2 tsp of the dried herb and infuse 10-15 minutes, drink x 3 a day.

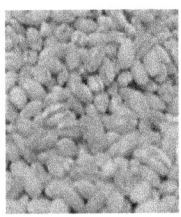

Barley (*Hordeum vulgare*) A body building grain good for wasting or debility, diuretic, mild relaxant for chest, barley water is used for kidney problems.

Recipe for Barley Water:

½ cup of whole barley
5 cups of water
¼ of a Cinnamon stick
Grated Ginger
Freshly squeezed lemon juice.

Place the whole barley, water, the cinnamon stick, some grated ginger in a pan and simmer for 20 minutes. After cooling, strain the mixture and add fresh lemon juice for extra flavour. Dosage: Drink 1-3 cups daily.
http://www.herbs-hands-healing.co.uk/drinks/barleywater.html

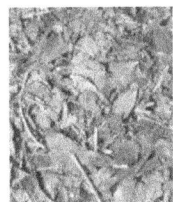

Bilberry (*Vaccinium myrtillus*) Soothes stomach upsets, sore throats, and urinary infections. A mouthwash can be made for ulcers & throat inflammations. Used for conditions of the eye.

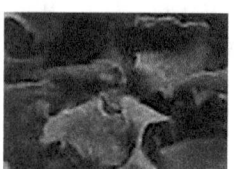 **Bladderwrack** *(Fucus vesiculous)* Anti-hypothyroid, anti-rheumatic. Used in treatment of underactive thyroid glands and goitre. Helpful in reducing weight. Provides relief for rheumatism, rheumatoid arthritis, internally, and externally when applied to inflamed joints. Dosage: Pour a cup of boiling water onto 2-3 tsp of dried herb, steep 10 minutes, drink x 3 a day.

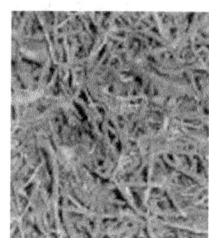 **Blue Cohosh** *(Caulophyllum thalictroides)* Uterine tonic, emmenagogue, anti-spasmodic, anti-rheumatic. Used in pregnancy when threat of miscarriage, eases false labour pains, Use just before birth, ensures an easy delivery. Used to bring on suppressed menstruation, anti-spasmodic for colic, Asthma, nervous coughs, eases rheumatic pain. Dosage: Put 1 tsp dried root in a cup of water, bring to boil, simmer 10 minutes drink x 3 a day.

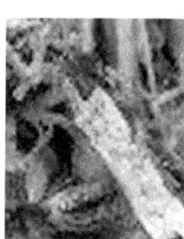 **Boneset** *(Eupatorium perfoliatum)* Used as a Diaphoretic, Febrifuge, Laxative, Stomachic, Stimulates appetite, anti-spasmodic, relaxes mucous membranes. Hepatic. Eases fevers, muscle aches of the flu; promotes sweating. Used in treatment of muscular rheumatism. **Caution: Is toxic in large doses or if taken over a long period of time.** Dosage: Pour a cup of boiling water onto 1-2 tsp of dried herb, infuse 10 -15 minutes. During fevers, flu, drink every half hour.

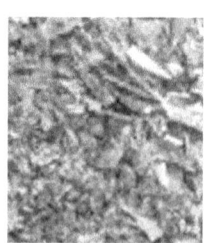 **Borage** *(Borago officinalis)* Reduces fever, coughs, sore throats, colds, decongestant for the lungs, expel poisons due to insect stings, itch, ringworms, scabs, sores, ulcers, a gargle for sores in the mouth and throat, loosens phlegm, used to restore vitality after illness. Externally, a poultice of leaves applied to inflamed swellings. Used in bath bombs to

nurture skin.

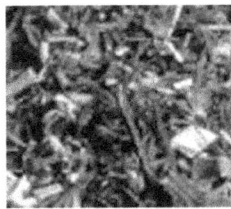 **Broom** *(Sarothamnus scoparius)* Cardioactive diuretic, hypertensive, peripheral vasoconstrictor, astringent. Remedy for a weak heart and low blood pressure. Increases efficiency of each stroke of the heart, used where water retention occurs because of heart weakness and for heavy menstruation. **Caution: Do not use Broom in pregnancy or hypertension.** Dosage: Pour a cup of boiling water onto 1 teaspoon of dried herb and infuse 10-15 minutes drink x 3 a day.

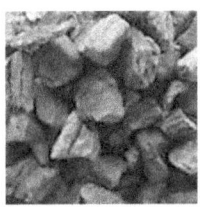 **Burdock** *(Arctium lappa)* Alternative, diuretic, bitter. Treatment of dry and scaly skin, such as psoriasis, dry Eczema, rheumatic conditions, aids digestion, appetite. Anorexia Nervosa, aids kidney function, cystitis, removes imbalance of skin problems, dandruff. Used as a compress or poultice externally for wounds, ulcers. Dosage: Put 1 tsp of root in a cup of water, bring to boil, simmer 10-15 minutes. Drink x 3 a day.

 **Caynenne Pepper** *(Capsicum minimum)* Used extensively by Mayan and Aztec. Nourishes the heart, removes plaque from the arteries, help rebuild flesh destroyed or harmed by frostbite, heal hemorrhoids, re-build stomach tissue, heals stomach ulcers. Good for circulation, equalizes blood pressure, used for gall bladder. Antifungal. Used as a rubefacient for lumbago, rheumatic pains. Dosage: Pour a cup of boiling water onto ½ to 1 tsp of Cayenne, infuse for 10 minutes. A tablespoon of this infusion should be mixed with hot water and drunk when needed.

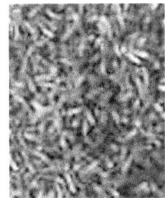 **Caraway** *(Carum carvi)* Aromatic, stimulant and carminative, expectorant, emmenagogue, galactagogue, astringent. Used for dyspepsia, pleasant stomachic. Used as a flavouring agents. For flatulent indigestion, use 1 to 4 drops of the essential oil of Caraway given on a lump of sugar, or in a teaspoonful of water. One ounce of the

bruised seeds infused for 6 hours in a pint of cold water used as a Caraway julep for infants, from 1 to 3 teaspoonfuls being given for a dose. The powder of the seeds, made into a poultice, will also take away bruises. Dosage: Pour a cup of boiling water onto 1 teaspoon of freshly crushed seeds; infuse 10 -15 minutes, drink x 3 a day.

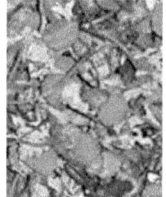

Chamomile Flower *(Anthemis nobilis)* Anti-spasmodic, carminative, anti-inflammatory, analgesic, antiseptic, vulnerary. Helps digestion, gastritis, gentle sedative, coughs, colds, poor skin, and is used as a liver tonic. Dosage: Pour a cup of boiling water onto 2 teaspoons of dried leaves, infuse 5-10 minutes. Should be drunk after meals for digestive problems, can be used as a mouthwash for gingivitis, For a steam bath, half a cup of flowers boiled in 2 litres water, cover your head with a towel and inhale the steam.

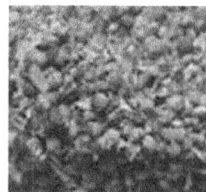

Chasteberry *(Vitex agnus-castus)* Known as a remedy used by women for hormone imbalance and menopause. Agnus castus is usually taken as a single dose first thing in the morning for both PMT (PMS) and menopause. Tonic for reproductive organs. Dosage: Pour cup of boiling water onto 1 teaspoon of ripe berries, infuse 10-15 minutes drink x 3 a day.

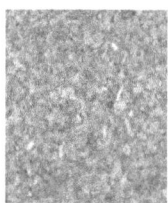

Celery Seed *(Apium graveolens)* Traditional remedy for nervous stomach, diuretic, carminative, mild tranquillizer used to relieve arthritic pain. **Caution: Can cause increased risk of sunburn in people who take prescription ACE inhibitors to control high blood pressure.**

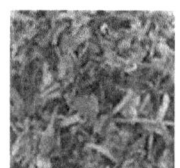

Chickweed Herb *(Stellaria media)* Anti-rheumatic, vulnerary, emollient. Dosage: Pour a cup of boiling water onto 2 tsp dried herbs, infuse 5 minutes. Drink x 3 a day. Chickweed may be made into an ointment, or used as a poultice. A strong infusion can be made and put into bath water. If being used for children for eczema internally, ¼ dose for children under 6, 1/2 dose for children 6-12.

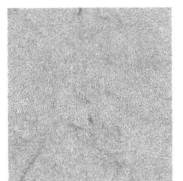

Cinnamon Powder *(Cinnamomum zeylanicum)* Eases stomach pains, colds, flu & digestive problems, athlete's foot. Strong antiseptic. Caution: Avoid taking large amounts during pregnancy. The German Commission E monograph suggests 1/2 -3/4 (2-4 grams of the powder per day). A tea can be prepared from the powdered herb by boiling 1/2 tsp (2-4 grams of the powder) for ten to fifteen minutes, cooling and then drinking.

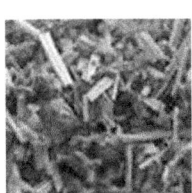

Cleavers *(Galium aperine)* Diuretic, alternative, anti-inflammatory, tonic, astringent, anti-neoplastic. Tonic for lymphatic system, Tonsillitis, adenoid. Psoriasis. Dosage: Pour a cup of boiling water onto 2-3 tsp of dried herb and infuse 10-15 minutes. Drink x 3 a day.

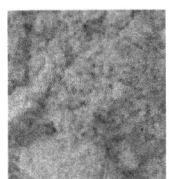

Clove *(Syzygium aromaticum)* Essential oil is used as an anodyne (painkiller) for dental emergencies, **Caution: Do not use long term as it can cause gum damage.** Carminative. Clove oil is used for acne, pimples, severe burns, skin irritations and to reduce the sensitiveness of skin. Used internally as a tea and topically as an oil for hypotonic muscles, including for multiple sclerosis.

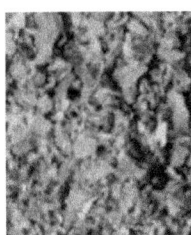

Coltsfoot *(Tussilago farfara)* Eases bronchitis coughs, & sore throats. Relaxing, expectorant, anti-tussive, demulcent, anti-catarrhal, diuretic. Pour a cup of boiling water onto 1-2 tsp of dried flowers and infuse for 10 minutes. Drink x 3 day.

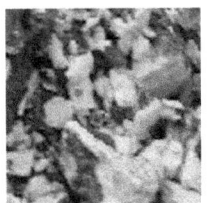

Comfrey Root *(Symphytum officinale)* Vulnerary, demulcent, astringent, expectorant. Used for gastric, duodenal ulcers, hiatus hernia, ulcerative colitis. **Caution: Do not use in deep wounds as it causes it to close too quickly before healed.** Used for Bronchitis, irritable cough. Used as a poultice in wounds and fractures. Dosage: 1-3 tsp. of dried herb in a cup of water, bring to boil, let simmer 10-15 minutes. Drink 3 times a day.

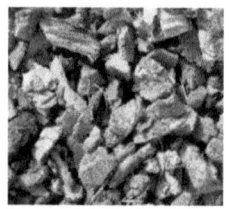

Cramp Bark (*Viburnum opulus*) Anti-spasmodic, sedative, astringent. Relaxer of muscular tension and spasm, ovarian, uterine muscle problems, used in treatment of large blood loss in periods and menopause. Dosage: Put 2 teaspoon of dried bark, into cup of water and bring to boil. Simmer for 10-15 minutes Drink x 3 a day.

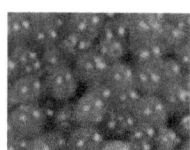

Cranberry (*Vaccinium oxycoccos*) Juice inhibits bacterial attachment to the bladder and urethra contains antioxidants that may help protect against heart disease, cancer and other diseases. Used in the prevention of ulcers, which are linked to stomach cancer and acid reflux disease.

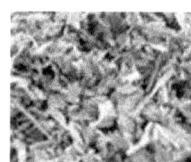

Damiana (*Turnera aphrodisiaca*) Nerve tonic, anti-depressant, urinary antiseptic, laxative. Remedy for nervous system, traditional aphrodisiac, used as an anti-depressant, anxiety as well as anxiety and depression with sexual difficulties, used to strengthen the male sexual system

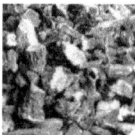

Dandelion Root *(Taraxacum officinale)* Diuretic, cholagogue, anti-rheumatic, laxative, tonic. Leaf-diuretic, source of potassium, used in water retention due to heart problems. Gentle tonic for liver function. Used in inflammation, congestion of liver and gallbladder, used in muscular rheumatism, general tonic. Dosage: Put 2 - 3 teaspoon of root in cup of water, bring to boil, gentle simmer 10-15 minutes, drink x 3 a day.

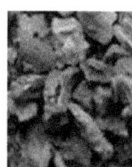

Devil's Claw *(Harpagophytum procumbrens)* Anti-inflammatory, anodyne, hepatic. Used in arthritis treatment, inflammation of joints, used in liver and gallbladder treatments. Dosage: ½ to 1 teaspoon in a cup of water, simmer 10-15 minutes, drink x 3 a day.

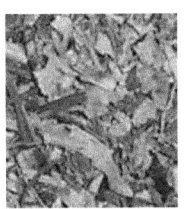

Echinacea Purpurea Root *(Echinacea angustifolia)* Anti-microbial, alterative. Used in treatment of boils, septicaemia, useful in infections of laryngitis, tonsillitis, catarrhal nose and throat, mouthwash for pyorrhoea, gingivitis, externally speed the healing of septic sores and cuts. Dosage, 1-2 tsp of root in one cup of water, bring to boil, let simmer for 10-15 minutes, drink x 3 a day.

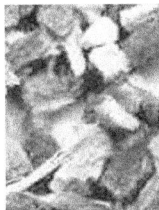

Elecampane *(Inula helenium)* Expectorant, anti-tussive, diaphoretic, stomachic, anti-bacterial. Treatment irritating bronchial coughs, lung tonic, bronchitis or emphysema, Asthma, bronchitic asthma, tuberculosis. Dosage: Pour a cup of cold water onto 1 teaspoon of shredded root, let stand 8-12 hours, heat up and take hot x 3 a day.

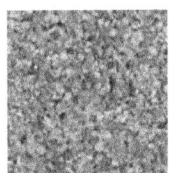

Elder *(Sambucus nigra)* Bark: purgative, emetic, diuretic, Leaves externally emollient and vulnerary, internally, purgative, expectorant, diuretic and diaphoretic, Flowers: Diaphoretic, anti-catarrhal, Berries: Diaphoretic, diuretic, laxative. Leaves used for bruises, sprains, wounds and chilblains, ointment for tumours, flowers treatment of colds and influenza, Hayfever, Sinusitis. Dosage: Pour a cup of boiling water onto 2 teaspoon of blossoms, leave to infuse for 10 minutes, drink x 3 a day.

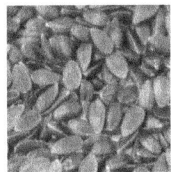

Ephedra *(Ephedra sinica)* Vasodilator, hypertensive, circulatory stimulant, anti-allergic. Treatment of asthma, relieves spasms in bronchial tubes, bronchitis, whooping cough, reduces allergic reactions, Hayfever, low blood pressure, circulatory insufficiency. Dosage: 1 - 2 tsp dried herb in one cup of water, bring to boil and simmer 10-15 minutes, drink x 3 a day.

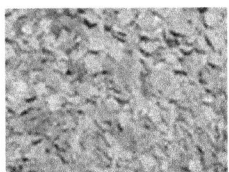

Eucalyptus *(Eucalyptus globulus)* Antiseptic, deodorant, antispasmodic, febrifuge, expectorant, stimulant, reduces blood sugar levels, vermifuge, aromatic, secretolytic, rubefacient, decongestant. Used in treatment of Asthma, upper respiratory congestion, bronchitis. **Caution: In large doses**

the oil is irritant to the kidneys, and it should not be taken internally, other than in lozenges. Used as a vapour bath or chest rub for asthma and other respiratory complaints, pyorrhoea and for burns, prevents infection. Eradicates lice and fleas. Used on purulent wounds and ulcers. Diluted in sunflower oil, for cold sores or used as an massage oil for painful joints. A cold extract made from the leaves is helpful for indigestion and for intermittent fever. In traditional Australian Aboriginal medicine the leaves are used in poultices for any type of wound and inflammation.

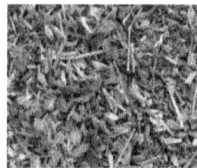

Eyebright *(Euphrasia officinalis)* Anti-catarrhal, astringent, anti-inflammatory. Remedy of mucous membrane, internally for anti-catarrhal, Sinusitis, for eyes, acute or chronic inflammation, stinging, weeping eye, sensitivity to light, use as compress, taken internally for conjunctivitis, blepharitis. Dosage: Infuse a cup of boiling water onto 1 teaspoon of dried herb and infuse 5-10 minutes, drink x 3 a day. For compress, place a teaspoon of dried herb in half a litre water, boil ten minutes, let cool, moisten a compress, in the lukewarm liquid, wring out and place over eyes, leave compress for 15 minutes, repeat several times a day.

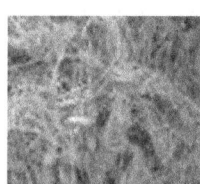

False Unicorn *(Chamaelirium luteum)* Uterine tonic, diuretic, anthelmintic, emetic. Normalizes hormones in both men and women, Tonic for reproductive system. Used in delayed or absent menstruation. For ovarian pain, helps prevent miscarriage, eases vomiting in pregnancy, **Caution: large dosages will cause vomiting.** Dosage: Put 1 - 2 teaspoons of root in cup of water, bring to boil, simmer gently for 15 minutes, drink x 3 a day.

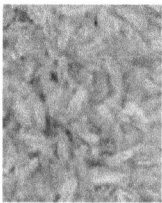

Fennel *(Foeniculum vulgare)* Carminative, aromatic, anti-spasmodic, stimulant, galactogogue, rubefacient, expectorant. Stomach and intestinal remedy for flatulence, colic, stimulates digestion and appetite, calming effect on bronchitis and coughs. Used as a flavouring, increases flow of milk in nursing mothers. Externally the oil is used for muscular and rheumatic pains. As an infusion it treats conjunctivitis and inflammation of eyelids as a compress. Dosage: Pour a cup of boiling water onto 1 - 2 teaspoonful of lightly crushed seeds, infuse for 10 minutes drink x 3 a day. For flatulence, drink half an hour before meals.

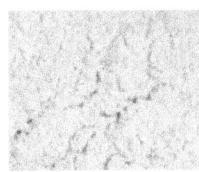

Fennugreek (*Trigonella foenum-graecum*) Anti-inflammatory, Antiseptic, Expectorant. Natural breast enlargement supplement. increase sexual stimulation, balance blood sugar levels and balance hormone levels to aid in treating PMS and menopause. Aphrodisiac. Contains Vitamins A and C, plus iron and phosphorous. Fenugreek is a blood, lymph and kidney tonic, and rids the body of toxins. Used to treat weakness, anaemia, infections, Sinusitis. **Caution: Should not be taken in pregnancy or with Glipizide, Heparin, Ticlopidine, Warfarin. Has a beneficial effect when taking Insulin.**

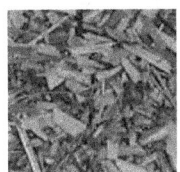

Feverfew (*Tanacetum parthenium*) Anti-inflammatory, vasodilatory, relaxant, digestive bitter, uterine stimulant. Used in treatment of migraine headaches, arthritis. Painful periods, sluggish menstral flow. **Caution: Should not be used in pregnancy. Fresh leaves can cause mouth ulcers.** Dosage equivalent of oneleaf taken 1-3 times a day.

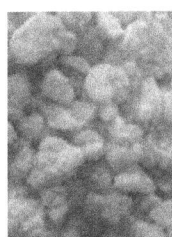

Frankincense (*Boswellia serrata*) Used in incense as well as in perfumes. Used in Ayurvedic medicine to treat arthritis, healing wounds, strengthening female hormone system, purifying atmosphere. Used in the treatment of Crohn's disease, ulcerative colitis, and osteoarthritis. Burning Frankincense repels mosquitoes.

Garlic Powder (*Allium sativum*) Antiseptic, anti-vial, diaphoretic, cholagogue, hypotensive, antispasmodic. Used for respiratory problems, earaches, bacterial infections, sore throats, colds, fevers, abscesses and injuries. Can be used in treatments for ear, skin and muscular conditions, infused in carrier oils and taken internally for worms, food poisoning, colds and flu, reduces blood pressure and blood cholesterol when taken over time. Used externally for treatment of ringworm and threadworm.

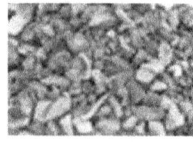 **Gentian** *(Gentiana lutea)* Bitter, gastric stimulant, cholagogue. Used for lack of appetite, sluggishness of the digestive system, dyspepsia, flatulence. Dosage: Put 1/2 teaspoonful of shredded root in a cup of water and boil for 5 minutes. Drink warm 15-30 minutes before meals and for acute stomach pains.

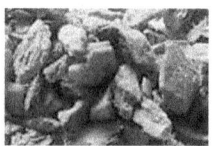 **Ginger** *(Zingiber officinale)* Stimulant, carminative, rubelacient, diaphoretic. Used to treat bad circulation, chilblains, cramp. Used in fevers, dyspepsia, flatulence, colic, as a gargle for sore throats, externally for fibrositis and muscle sprains. Dosage: Pour a cup of boiling water onto 1 tsp of fresh root, infuse five minutes. For powder, put 1 1/2 teaspoonful in a cup of water, bring to boil and simmer for 5-10 minutes, drink when needed.

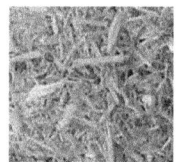 **Gingseng** *(Panax ginseng)* Adaptogen, aphrodisiac, anti-depressive, improves physical and mental performance. Used to raise low blood pressure, Depression due to debility, exhaustion. **Caution: May produce headaches in some people.** Dosage: Put 1/2 teaspoonful of powder in a cup of water, bring to boil, simmer gently for 10 minutes. Drink x 3 a day.

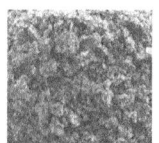 **Flaxseed** *(Linum usitatissimum)* Demulcent, anti-tussive, laxative, emollient, Used in chest infections, poultice in pleurisy, pulmonary condition, boils, carbuncles, shingles and psoriasis, purgative for constipation. Dosage: Pour a cup of boiling water onto 2 - 3 teaspoonful of dried herb and infuse for 10-15 minutes, drink in morning and evening.

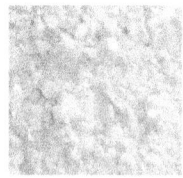 **Fullers Earth** *(Green Clay or Bentonite (Magnesium Aluminium Silicate)* Used in treatment of leg ulcers because of its drawing and sterilizing action. Used externally as a skin cleanser, defoliator. For internal cleansing put one tsp of clay in a glass of spring water, leave to stand overnight, stir the mixture the next morning and drink before breakfast.

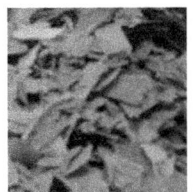 **Gingko Biloba** Anti-inflammatory, Antioxidant, Improves blood flow, Strengthens blood vessels. Relaxes the lungs, circulatory system tonic, vasodilator. Used in treatments for sexual function in men and women, circulation, mental function, eyesight, impotence, vertigo, tinnitus, male enhancement, Acrocyanosis, Alzheimer's, Asthma, cerebral atherosclerosis, cochlear deafness, dementia, depression, diabetes related nerve damage and poor circulation, diabetic retinopathy, improving circulation to the brain in the elderly, leg ulcers, macular degeneration, menopause, multiple sclerosis, Parkinson's Disease, PMS, Raynaud's disease, Sinusitis, strokes, thrombosis, tinnitus, varicose veins and vertigo. Dosage: Pour 1 cup of boiling water over 1 tsp of dried herb, infuse 10-15 minutes, drink x 3 a day.

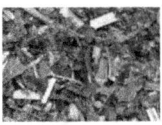 **Goldenrod** (*Solidago virgaurea*) Anti-inflammatory, anti-microbial. Used in treatment of the inflammation of the bladder or urinary tract, kidney stones, influenza, upper respiratory congestion, arthritis, periodontal disease and gastrointestinal disorders. Dosage: Pour 1 cup of boiling water over 1 tsp of dried herb, infuse 10-15 minutes, drink x 3 a day.

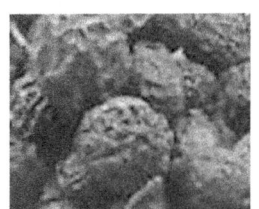 **Hawthorne Berries** (*Crataegus oxyacanthoides*) Cardiac tonic, hypotensive. Remedy of heart and circulatory system. Normalizes heart function in a gentle way, arteriosclerosis, angina pectoris, varicose veins and ulcers. Dosage: Pour a cup of boiling water onto 2 teaspoonfuls of berries and leaves, infuse 20 minutes, drink x 3 a day, can be used over a long period.

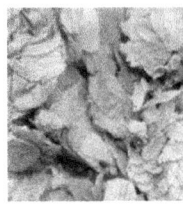 **Hops** (*Humulus lupulus*) Sedative, hypnotic, antiseptic, astringent. Relaxes central nervous system, treatment of insomnia, tension anxiety, indigestion, mucous colitis. **Caution: Do not use in cases of severe Depression.** Dosage: Pour a cup of boiling water onto 1 teaspoonful of dried flowers and infuse for 10-15 minutes, a cup should be drunk at night to induce sleep.

45

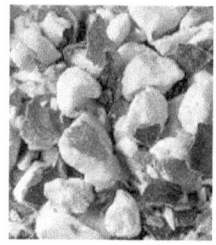

Horsechestnut *(Aesculus hippocastanum)*
Astringent, circulatory tonic. Strengthens
and/tones veins. Used internally to aid body in
treatment of phlebitis, inflammation of veins,
varicosity, haemorrhoids, externally as a lotion.
Dosage: Pour a cup of boiling water onto 1-2 tsp
of dried fruit, leave to infuse for 10-15 minutes
drink x 3 a day or use to make a lotion.

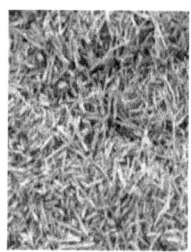

Horsetail *(Equisetum arvense)* Astringent, diuretic,
vulnerary. Astringent for genito-urinary system,
reducing haemorrhage, healing wounds, mild
diuretic, inflamed/ benign enlargement of prostrate,
ease pain of rheumatism, chilblains. Dosage: Pour
a cup of boiling water onto 2 tsp of dried herb,
infuse for 15-20 minutes x 3 a day.

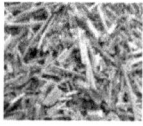

Hyssop *(Hyssopus officinalis)* Anti-spasmodic,
expectorant, diaphoretic, sedative, carminative. Coughs,
bronchitis, chronic catarrh, common cold, nervine,
anxiety, petit mal (epilepsy). Dosage: Pour a cup of
boiling water onto-1 - 2 tsp of dried herb, leave to infuse for 10-15
minutes, drink x 3 a day.

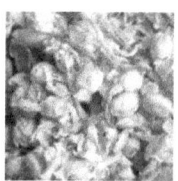

Jasmine *(Jasmine officinalis)* Anti-depressant,
antiseptic, aphrodisiac, anti-spasmodic, cicatrisant,
expectorant, galactagogue, parturient, sedative and
uterine. **Caution: Do not use during pregnancy**.
Eases coughs, sore eyes, tension, mild-
antidepressant. Uplift your Spirits Tea (Herbmoonhollow.com) 2 oz
Lemon Balm, Ginkgo, Nettles, Jasmine Flowers, Hawthorn, Dandelion
Root, Liquorice Root, Lavender. Use 1 tsp per cup of boiling water.

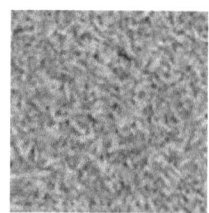

Lavender *(Lavendula angustifolia)* Antiseptic,
analgesic, anti-convulsant, anti-depressant, anti-
rheumatic, anti-spasmodic, anti-inflammatory,
antiviral, bactericide, carminative, cholagogue,
cicatrisant, cordial, cytophylactic, decongestant,
deodorant, diuretic, emmenagogue, hypotensive,

nervine, rubefacient, sedative, sudorific and vulnerary. Calming effect on the nerves, relieving tension, depression, panic, hysteria and nervous exhaustion in general and is effective for headaches, migraines and insomnia, bronchitis, asthma, colds, laryngitis, halitosis, throat infections and whooping cough and helps the digestive system deal with colic, nausea, vomiting and flatulence. Relieves pain when used for rheumatism, arthritis, lumbago and muscular aches and pains. Skin conditions: abscesses, acne, oily skin, boils, burns, sunburn, wounds, psoriasis, lice, insect bites, stings and also acts as an insect repellent. Dosage: Pour a cup of boiling water onto-1-2 tsp of dried herb, leave to infuse for 10-15 minutes, drink x 3 a day. A drop of lavender oil can be put on a sugar cube for relief for migraines.

Lady's Mantle *(Alchemilla vulgaris)* Astringent, diuretic, anti-inflammatory, vulnerary. Eases period pains, excessive bleeding, used in treatment of menopause, used internally in diarrhoea and externally for cuts and wounds. Dosage: Pour a cup of boiling water onto 2 tsp of dried herb, steep for 10-15 minutes drink x 3 a day.

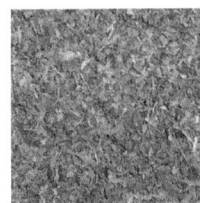

Lemon Balm *(Melissa officinalis)* Helps to reduce excessive blood pressure. Calming and regulating effect on the menstrual cycle, ease of menstrual cramps and alleviation of scanty menstruation. Calmative for digestion difficulties, flatulence, antiviral and anti-histamine properties. Dosage: Pour a cup of boiling water onto 2 tsp of dried herb, steep for 10-15 minutes drink x 3 a day.

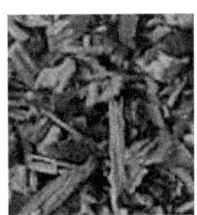

Liquorice Root *(Glycyrrhiza glabra)* Expectorant, demulcent, anti-inflammatory, adrenal agent, anti-spasmodic, mild laxative. Used in treatment of adrenal gland conditions, Addison's disease, bronchial conditions, bronchitis, coughs, peptic ulceration, gastritis and ulcers, abdominal colic. Dosage: Put 1/2 - 1 tsp of root into a cup of water, bring to boil and simmer for 10-15 minutes, drink x 3 a day.

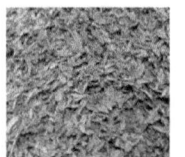 **Marjoram** *(Origanum marjorana linnaeus)* Used to treat insomnia, headaches, colds, Asthma, bronchitis, muscular tension, menstrual cramps, rheumatism, high blood pressure and constipation. **Caution: Avoid during pregnancy.** Dosage: Pour a cup of boiling water onto 2 tsp of dried herb, steep for 10-15 minutes drink x 3 a day.

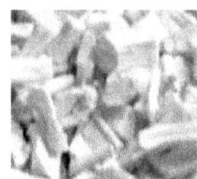 **Marshmallow Root** *(Althaea officinalis)* Root: demulcent, diuretic, emollient, vulnerary, Leaf, Demulcent, expectorant, diuretic, emollient. Root used for digestive and skin problems, leaf is used for lungs and urinary system. Inflammation of the mouth, gastritis, peptic ulcer, enteritis, colitis. Root is used for bronchitis, respiratory catarrh, irritating coughs, urethritis, urinary gravel leaf is used. Externally root is used for varicose veins, ulcers, abscesses and boils. A compress or poultice can be made. Dosage: Put root into a cup of water, boil gently 10-15 minutes, drink x 3 a day. Leaves: Pour boiling water onto 1-2 tsp of dried leaf, infuse 10 minutes, drink x 3 a day.

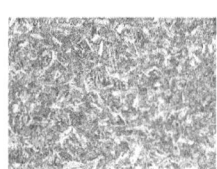 **Meadowsweet** *(Filipendula ulmaria)* Anti-rheumatic, anti-inflammatory, stomachic, antacid, antemetric, astringent. Protects and soothes digestive tract, reduces acidity, eases nausea, used to treat heartburn, hyperactivity, gastritis, peptic ulceration, reduces fever, relieves pain of rheumatism in muscles and joints. Dosage: Pour a cup of boiling water onto 1-2 tsp of dried herb and leave to infuse for 10-5 minutes, drink x 3 a day.

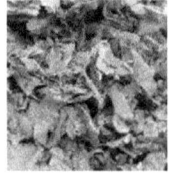 **Milk thistle** *(Carduus marianus)* Liver function stimulant, Detoxification, Gallstones, High cholesterol, Liver tonic. Used to treat morning sickness, motion sickness, lessens varicose veins, haemorrhoids caused by poor circulation during pregnancy. Encourages good milk production, calming. Used in treatment of **acne and psoriasis.** Dosage: Pour a cup of boiling water onto 1-2 tsp of dried herb and leave to infuse for 10-5 minutes, drink x 3 a day.

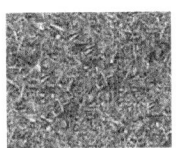 **Motherwort** *(Leonurus cardiac)* Sedative, emmenagogue, anti-spasmodic, cardiac tonic. Used to treat uterine and menstrual, heart and circulation conditions. Relaxing tonic for menopause, false labour pains, tonic for heart, delayed and suppressed menstruation, over-rapid heart beats, palpitations. Dosage: Pour a cup of boiling water onto 1-2 tsp of dried herb and leave to infuse for 10-15 minutes, drink x 3 a day.

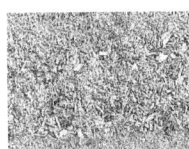 **Mugwort** *(Artemisia vulgaris)* Bitter tonic, stimulant, nervine tonic, emmenagogue. Used as a flavouring, digestive stimulant, aids digestion, mild nervine action aids in Depression, eases tension, used to aid normal menstrual flow. Dosage: Infusion: Pour a cup of boiling water onto 1-2 tsp of herb, infuse 10-15 minutes in a covered container, drink x 3 a day.

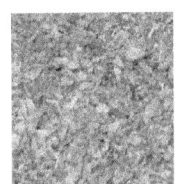 **Mullein** *(Verbascum thapsus)* Expectorant, demulcent, mild diuretic, mild sedative, vulnerary. Respiratory remedy, tones mucous membranes, reduces inflammation, and facilitates expectoration. Tones and normalizes chest. Bronchitis, anti-inflammatory, used in inflammation of the trachea. Externally used in olive oil to sooth and heal inflamed skin. Dosage: Pour a cup of boiling water onto 1-2 tsp of dried leaves or flowers, infuse for 10-15 minutes, drink x 3 a day.

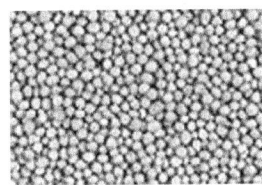 **Mustard** *(Sinapis alba)* Mustard plaster recipe : 4 tablespoons flour, 1 tablespoon dry mustard, add hot water and make into a dry paste. Apply onto a cloth, fold over twice and place on chest or sore area for 15 minutes, then remove. Used for aches, sprains, and eliminating mucus from the lungs. Heals watery, oozing and chronic sores and boils.

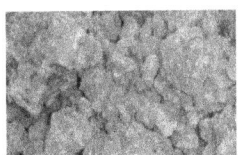 **Myrrh** *(Commiphora molmol)* Anti-microbial, astringent, carminative, anti-catarrhal, expectorant, vulnerary. Used in treatment of mouth ulcers, gingivitis, pyorrhoea, Pharyngitis, sinusitis, laryngitis, respiratory complaints, used to treat boils, glandular fever, brucellosis, common cold, externally for wounds and abrasions. Dosage: Powder and pour a cup of boiling water onto 1-2 tsp of powder and infuse 10-15 minutes drink x 3 a day.

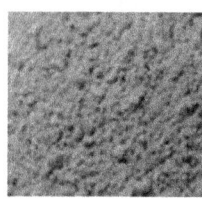

Neem *(Azadirachta indica)* Anthelmintic (parasites and worms), Antipyretic, Antiseptic, Emmenagogue. Used to treat, Arthritis, Bronchitis, Cough, Diabetes, Diuretic, Eczema, Erysipelas, Fever Jaundice, Leukorrhea, Lice. Malaria, Nausea, Obesity, Rheumatism, Scrofula, Skin diseases, Syphilis, Tetanus, Tumors, Urticaria Vomiting.

Caution: Pregnant and nursing mothers should not take Neem.
Dosage: Pour a cup of boiling water onto 1-2 tsp of dried herb, infuse for 10-15 minutes, drink x 3 a day.

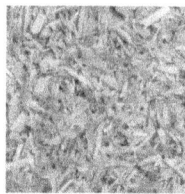

Oat Straw *(Avena sativa)* Used to treat nervous exhaustion and insomnia, rheumatic conditions, water retention, tobacco withdrawal, anxiety, and in the bath for skin conditions such as burns and eczema. Dosage: Pour a cup of boiling water onto 1-2 tsp of dried herb, infuse for 10-15 minutes, drink x 3 a day.

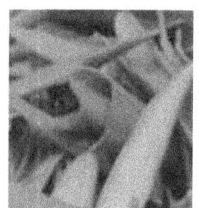

Olive Leaf *(Olea europaea)* Antiseptic, astringent, lowers fever, blood pressure, calming, used to treat kidney function. Antioxidant, used in heart and circulatory treatments. Leaf is drunk as a tea. Used to treat chronic fatigue, as an anti-viral and for colic . Dosage: Pour a cup of boiling water onto 1-2 tsp of dried herb, infuse for 10-15 minutes, drink x 3 a day. Externally olive oil is used as a carrier oil for herbs, such as balm of gilead and essential oils or for infused culinary oils.

Orris Root *(Iris florentina)* Used as a remedy for sore throats, colds, mild diuretic, has a violet-like scent and is used as a fixative for incense. It is a natural breath freshener, used in toothpastes, strengthens gums.

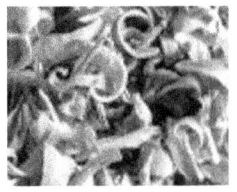

Orange Flowers (Bergamot)*(Citrus aurantium)* Bergamot is used as a tonic for stimulating a poor appetite and alleviating gas and indigestion, cystitis, thrush and itching. Sedative used for anxiety, depression and stress related conditions. Used in treatment of sore throats, tonsillitis, colds, flu and respiratory infections, oily skin, acne, spots, boils and herpes; and stress related skin problems such as Eczema and Psoriasis. Bergamot Tea: Infuse 1 teaspoon dried bergamot in 1 covered cup boiling water for fifteen minutes. Strain and add honey to flavor. **Caution: When using Bergamot Essential Oil do not expose skin to bright sunlight as it increases photosensitivity of the skin.**

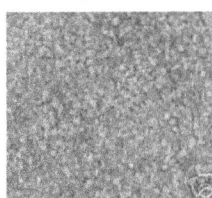

Orange Peel *(Citrus sinensis)* Used in teas for flavour and to aid with digestive problems and stimulate appetite. Used in cosmetics face masks to open pores, soaps, in potpourri for colour and scent. Used in love sachets and prosperity incenses. Chinese considered oranges symbols of luck and good fortune.

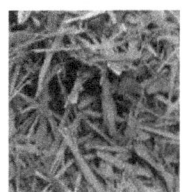

Pau D'arco *(Tabebuia avellanadae)* Used in treatment of Candida yeast infections, infectious diarrhoea, bladder infections, parasitic infections, cancer, diabetes, ulcers, gastritis, liver ailments, asthma, bronchitis, cystitis, prostatitis, ringworm, rheumatism, hernias, gonorrhea, syphilis, chlorosis, boils, wounds, as a "tonic and blood builder," viral respiratory infections, colds, flu, smoker's cough, warts and acne. Dosage: Pour a cup of boiling water onto 1-2 teaspoonfuls of herb infuse for 10 minutes. Drink x 3 a day.

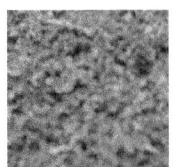

Parsley *(Petroselinum crispum)* Diuretic, Expectorant, Emmenagogue, Carminative, Aphrodisiac. Rich source of Vitamin C, used as diuretic, stimulates menstrual process. **Caution: Do not use Parsley in medicinal doses during Pregnancy**. Eases flatulence, colic. Dosage: Pour a cup of boiling water onto 1 teaspoonfuls of leaves or root and infuse for 5-10 minutes in a closed container. Drink x 3 a day.

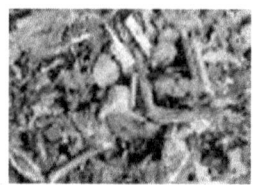

Passiflora *(Passiflora incarnate)* Sedative, hypnotic, anti-spasmodic, anodyne. Used to treat insomnia, Parkinson's disease, seizures and hysteria, nerve pain, neuralgia, shingles, Asthma with tension. Dosage: Pour a cup of boiling water onto 1 teaspoonful of dried herb and let infuse for 15 minutes. Drink a cup in the evening for sleeplessness, cup twice a day for easing of conditions.

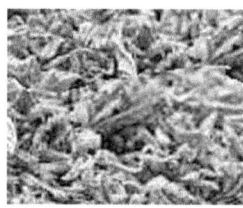

Penny Royal *(Mentha pulegium)* Carminative, Diaphoretic, Emmenogogue Antispasmodic, Mild Sedative, Sudorific, Stimulant, Aromatic, Abortifacient. Used in treatment of nausea & nervous conditions, headaches, menstrual cramps, PMS, pain, phlegm, gall bladder & respiratory disorders, jaundice, nausea, ulcers, consumption, dropsy, toothache, leprosy, whooping cough, convulsions, sores in the mouth, colic, snakebites, expel after-birth, sore gums, fainting, fever, & gout. Purifies the blood, relieves gas & stomach pain, stimulates uterine contractions. Used externally for skin eruptions, bruises, rashes, & itching. Dosage: Pour a cup of boiling water onto 1 heaped tsp. of dried herb and infuse for 10 minutes. **Caution: Do not be used during pregnancy-uterine stimulant, fetal damage may occur from the use of pennyroyal in any form. May cause severe kidney/liver damage used in excess of 2 ounces.**

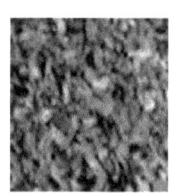

Peppermint *(Mentha piperita)* Carminative, Anti-spasmodic, Aromatic, Diaphoretic, Anti-emetic, Nervine, Antiseptic, Analgesic Inhibits mucous secretion temporarily, anti-spasmodic, relaxing on visceral muscles, anti-flatulence, stimulates bile and digestive juice secretion, relieves intestinal colic, dyspepsia, nausea, relieves vomiting during pregnancy, travel sickness, ulcerative colitis, Chrohn's disease. Treatment of fevers, colds, influenza, migraines, eases anxiety, tension, hysteria, painful periods, externally, relieves itching and inflammations. Dosage: Pour a cup of boiling water onto 1 heaped tsp. of dried herb, infuse for 10 minutes.

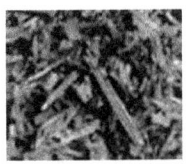

Plantain *(Plantago major)*Expectorant, demulcent, astringent, diuretic. Gentle expectorant, soothes inflamed, sore membranes, coughs, bronchitis, diarrhoea, haemorrhoids, cystitis with bleeding. Dosage: Pour a cup of boiling water onto 2 teaspoonful of dried herb and infuse for 10 minutes. Drink three times a day. Ointment can be made to treat cuts and haemorrhoids. Can be used in Lavender and Hops bags to promote sleep.

Pumice Powder *(Pumice)* Used in face cream base, soap base, shower gel base, foot scrubs and in Gardening Soaps.

Recipe for Gardeners Soap (Herbmoonhollow.com)

250 melt and pour soap base
2 mls tea tree essential oil
1 Tablespoon Ground Pumice Powder
1 Teaspoon sweet almond oil
Add colour of your choice if desired.
Melt the soap base and allow to cool slightly, add the sweet almond oil and stir gently add the powdered pumice and mix thoroughly, add the tea tree oil, pour into moulds and allow to set.

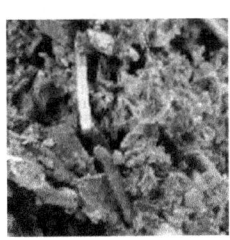

Raspberry Leaf *(Rubus idaeus)* Astringent, tonic refrigerant, parturient. Used in pregnancy to strengthen and tone the tissue of the womb, assists contractions checks haemorrhage during labour if drunk during pregnancy and during labour. Used to treat diarrhoea, leucorrhoea, eases mouth ulcers, bleeding gums, inflammations, as gargle for sore throats. Dosage: Pour a cup of boiling water onto 2 tsp of dried herb and infuse for 10-15 minutes, drink regularly.

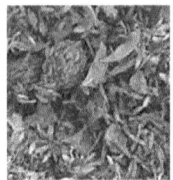 **Red Clover Leaf** *(Trifolium pratense)* Alternative, expectorant, antispasmodic. Used as a remedy for children's skin problems, such as Eczema, and Psoriasis, used in treatment of coughs, bronchitis, whooping cough. Dosage: Pour a cup of boiling water onto 1-3 teaspoonful of dried herb and infuse for 10-15 minutes, drink x 3 a day.

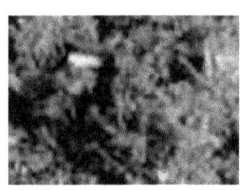 **Red Sage** *(Salvia officinalis)* Carminatives, spasmolytic, antiseptic, astringent, anti-hidrotic. Traditional remedy for inflammation of mouth, throat, tonsils, mucous membrane, used internally and as a mouthwash for inflamed gums, tongue, mouth ulcers, gargle for laryngitis, pharyngitis, tonsillitis and quinsy. Used in treatment of dyspepsia, reduces production of breast milk. As a compress for wounds, **Caution: Avoid during pregnancy.** Dosage: Pour a cup of boiling water onto 1-2 tsp of leaves and infuse for 10 minutes, drink three times a day. For mouthwash: Put 2 teaspoonfuls of leaves in half a litre of water, bring to boil, let stand covered for 15 minutes, gargle for 5-10 minutes several times a day.

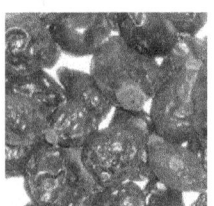 **Rosehips** *(Rosa Canina)* Antidepressant & anti-inflammatory. Rose hips are very high in Vitamin C. Rose hips also contain A, B, E, and K, organic acids and pectin, and have a high concentration of iron. Infused in oil can be used externally. Rose hips are very nourishing to the skin. Used in treatment of Rheumatism, Arthritis, shown to lessen use of painkillers in study done in Copenhagen. Also used in Potpourri.

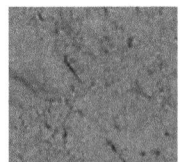 **Rosehips Powder** *(Rosa Canina)* Used in capsules, can be added to teas, creams.

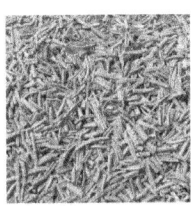

Rosemary *(Rosemarinus officinalis)* Carminative, aromatic, anti-spasmodic, anti-depressive, antiseptic, rubefacient, parasiticide. Circulatory and nervine stimulant, toning and calming on digestion, flatulence, dyspepsia, headache, depression, Externally used to ease muscular pain, sciatica and neuralgia. Used as a stimulant to the hair to prevent premature balding (essential oil) Dosage: Pour a cup of boiling water onto 1-2 teaspoonful of dried herb, leave to infuse in a covered container 10-15 minutes, drink x 3 a day.

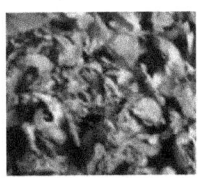

Rose Petals *(Rosa centifolia)* Rose tea is used to treat circulation and strengthens the heart the stomach, the liver and the retentive faculty. Red rose is used for fluxes, to prevent vomiting, tickling coughs and consumption. Sooths nerves, anti-depressant, calms anger, hangovers. Can be burned as incense, used in bath, potpourri and for decorations. Pour a cup of boiling water onto 1-2 teaspoonfuls of dried herb, leave to infuse in a covered container 10-15 minutes, drink x 3 a day.

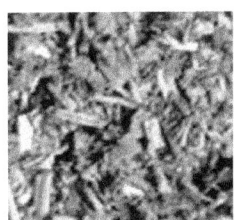

Rue *(Ruta graveolens)* Anti-spasmodic, emmenagogue, anti-tussive, aborifacient. Used to regulate menstrual periods **Caution: Avoid during pregnancy.** Relaxes smooth muscles in digestive system, spasmodic coughs, increases peripheral circulation, lowers elevated blood pressure. Fresh leaf chewed will relieve tension headaches, ease palpitations, anxiety. Dosage: Pour a cup of boiling water onto 1-2 teaspoonfuls of dried herb, infuse for 10-15 minutes, drink x 3 a day.

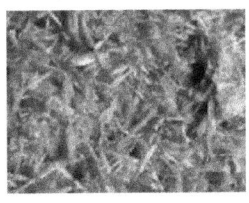

Safflower Petals *(Carthamus tinctorius)* Used in TCM to improve blood circulation. Anti-carcinogenic, Anti-inflammatory, Antioxidant. Used in breast cancer treatment. Oil is used in anti-tumor treatment of skin cancer. Used in soaps, salts and bath bombs or infused in oil and added to give a delicate red colour. Used as a natural dye to produce yellow or red dye and in potpourri. Dosage: Pour a cup of boiling water onto 1-2 teaspoonfuls of dried herb, infuse for 10-15 minutes, drink x 3 a day.

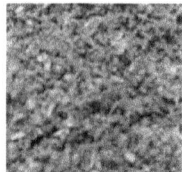 **Sage** (*Salvia officinalis*) Carminatives, spasmolytic, antiseptic, astringent, anti-hidrotic. Used to relieve mucous buildup. Eases mental exhaustion improves concentration. Used in lotion or salves for treating sores and skin eruptions and to stop bleeding cuts, for stomach complaints, diarrhea, gas, flu and colds. As a hair rinse, removes dandruff. For headaches, combine with peppermint, rosemary and wood betony. Regulates menstrual flow, decrease lactating milk, treats hot flashes. Dosage: Pour a cup of boiling water onto 1-2 teaspoonfuls of dried herb, infuse for 10-15 minutes, drink x 3 a day.

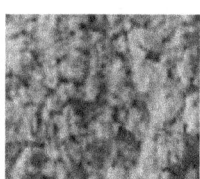 **Slippery Elm** (*Ulmus fulva*) Demulcent, emmolient, nutrient, astringent. Used to treat sensitive or inflamed mucous membrane in digestive system, IBS, gastritis, gastric or duodenal ulcer, enteritis, colitis, used as food during convalescence, diarrhoea, poultice of boils, abscesses, ulcers. Dosage: Use 1 part powdered bark to 8 parts water, mix powder in a little water to begin mixture, then add rest of water, bring to boil, simmer gently 10-15 minutes drink half a cup x 3 a day. For poultice mix powdered bark with enough boiling water to make a paste. For lozenges: melt honey first and then add powdered slippery elm, mix into a dough spread out onto clean surface and score with knife into sections, when set, wrap in cellophane.

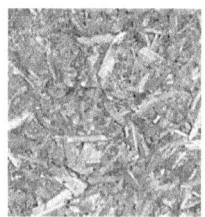 **St. John's Wort** *(Hypericum perforatum)* Nervine tonic, anti-inflammatory, astringent, vulnerary. Internally used as a sedative, restorative, pain-reducing for neuralgia, anxiety, tension, used for nervous debility, stress, in menopause for irritability and anxiety, fibrositis, sciatica, rheumatic pain, externally as an anti-inflammatory, speeds healing of wounds, bruises, varicose veins, mild burns, oil is used for healing of sunburn. Depression relief. (**Caution: Not to be used for severe depression**). Dosage: Pour a cup of boiling water onto 1-2 teaspoonfuls of dried

herb, infuse for 10-15 minutes.

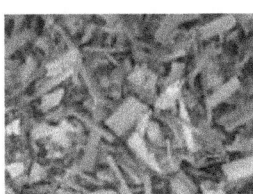

Sweet Violet (*Viola odorata*) Expectorant, alternative, anti-inflammatory, diuretic, anti-neoplastic, Used as a cough remedy, bronchitis, skin condition eczema, long term treatment of rheumatism, urinary infection, anti-cancer herb. Dosage: Pour a cup of boiling water onto 1 teaspoonful of herb, infuse for 10-15 minutes drink x 3 a day. Can be used in a muslin bag as a sleep pillow for a bad chest.

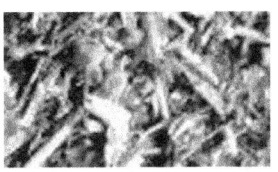

Tansy (*Tanacetum vulgare*) Anthelmintic, anti-parasitic, bitter, carminative, emmenagogue, aromatic, tonic, diaphoretic, vulnerary. Used for: scabies (external wash), digestive bitter, roundworm & threadworm. For intestinal worms it may be used with Wormwood & a carminative such as Chamomile, in conjunction with a purgative like Senna. Used to repel fleas, mix with crushed lavender buds and baking soda for a carpet freshener. **Caution: Do not use if pregnant. Do not take in large doses. Relaxing-Calming Baths** (herbmoon hollow) Make an infusion and add to bath water 2 tbsp each of, Rose Petals, Tansy, Raspberry Leaf, Valerian Root

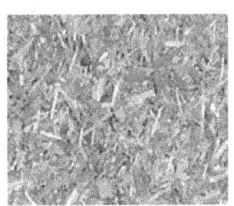

Thyme (*Thymus vulgaris*) Carminative, anti-microbial, anti-spasmodic, expectorant, astringent, mild anthelmintic. Used in treatment of indigestion, digestive system infections, treatment of laryngitis, tonsillitis, bronchitis, bronchitis, whooping cough, asthma, externally, antiseptic wash for cuts, sores and infect wounds. Dosage: Pour a cup of boiling water onto 2 teaspoonfuls of dried herb, infuse in a covered pot for 10 minutes, drink x 3 a day.

Tumeric (*Curcuma longa*) Anti-inflammatory, antioxidant, digestive, anti-bacterial Used in treatment of arthritis, digestive problems, IBS, and circulatory disorders. Used in Ayurvedic medicine as a digestive, circulatory and respiratory stimulant. It has also long been used to help cleanse the chakras. Dosage: 1.5 – 3 g of the herb to be taken daily as needed in powder or capsule form.

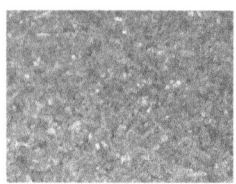 **Valerian Root** *(Valerian officinalis)* Sedative, hypnotic, anti-spasmodic, hypotensive, carminative. Relaxing nervine, reduces tension, anxiety, hysterical states. Relief of cramp and intestinal colic, cramps and pains of periods, migraine, rheumatic pain. Dosage: Pour a cup of boiling water onto 1-2 teaspoonfuls of root, infuse for 10-15 minutes, drink as needed.

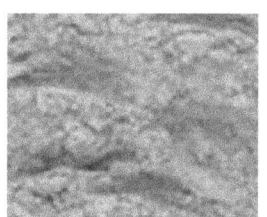 **Wheatgrass Powder** *(Triticum aestivum)* Used to treat the digestive system, diabetes and heart disease, constipation, abdominal coldness and spasmic pain, constipation and cough. Anti-cancer properties, detoxify heavy metals from the bloodstream, help make menopause more manageable, promotes general well-being. Dosage: 1/2 to 4 teaspoons per day added to smoothies, water, dips or can be taken in capsule form.

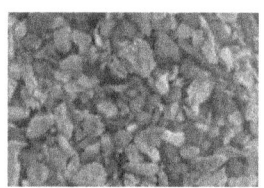 **Wild Yam** *(Dioscorea villosa)* Natural pain reliever, PMS. reduces menstrual cramping, relieves symptoms related to menopause, decreases water retention and alleviates nausea caused by pregnancy. Used to treat arthritis, rheumatism and muscle spasms, eases digestion, reduction of cholesterol and blood pressure levels. Relax muscles and help reduce inflammation.

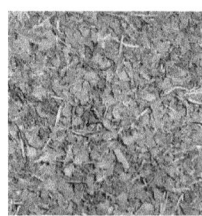 **Wood Betony** *(Stachys betonica)* Sedative, nervine tonic, bitter. Strengthens the central nervous system, used to treat anxiety, tension, eases headaches, neuralgia. Dosage: Pour a cup of boiling water onto 1-2 teaspoonfuls of dried herb, infuse for 10-15 minutes drink x 3 a day.

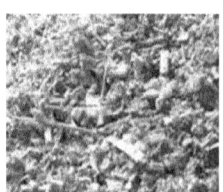 **Wormwood** *(Artemesia absinthium)* Eases bruising, sprains; use as a muscle relaxant, digestive system, liver and bladder ailments. It promotes menstruation and will help with menstrual cramps. Remedies for worms.

**Caution: Do not give to small children, and use only in very
small quantities for very short periods of time**

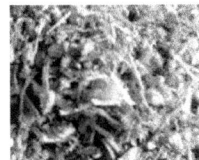 **Yarrow Herb** *(Achillea millefolium)* Diaphoretic,
hypotensive, astringent, diuretic, antiseptic. Used in
treatment of fevers, lowers blood pressure, stimulates
digestion, urinary antiseptic, used for cystitis, used
externally to heal wounds. Dosage: Pour a cup of
boiling water onto 1-2 teaspoonfuls of dried herb and infuse for 10-15
minutes, drink x 3 a day. For a fever, drink hourly.

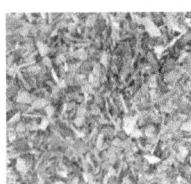 **Yerba Mate** *(Ilex paraguariensis)* Stimulates nervous
system, used to treat headaches, migraines, fatigue, mild
depression, boosts the immune system. Compress for
Aching Joints and Bones: Meadowsweet, Yerba Mate
and Wormwood. Pour 1 cup of boiling water over 1/4
oz each herb, cool, make a compress, apply to aching
part.

7 MAKING HERBAL PREPARATIONS

Making herbal preparations requires a clean space with a hat and coat worn to prevent contamination. Any Manufacturer Safety Sheets, like for Essential Oils should be nearby. Safety glasses are also recommended especially when using Peppermint essential oil or making soaps and gloves or tongs should be used to protect hands.

A log should be kept of ingredients used and suppliers and when the product was made. INCI names must be used when making labels, I put the common name as well and all ingredients must be listed. A batch number and expiry date must appear on the labelling, as well as a weight or volume. Product and public liability insurance must be had when selling to the public. (Examples: Aromantic, MAIB, Towergate)

Making Infused Oils

Making an infused oil using almond *(Prunus amygdalis dulcus)*, Grapeseed *(Vitis vinifera)*, Jojoba *(Simmondsia chinensis)*, Olive *(Olea europaea)*, Sunflower *(Helianthus annuus)*, Sesame *(Sesamum indicum)*, Avocado oil *(Persea gratissima)* or other oil with the dried or fresh herb, cook slowly for 5 hours, a slow cooker just for herbal products is ideal.

For making infused rose hip oil, put rose hips in a mortar and pestle and open then up before putting them in the oil. It is also possible to infuse oils in the sun for two weeks, shaking the bottle every couple of days. Add an essential oils used last to prevent them from evaporating and drain the possible to infuse oils in the sun for two weeks, shaking the bottle every couple of days. Add any essential oils used last to prevent them from evaporating and drain the herbs from the oil when cool and decant into amber bottle. Vitamin E Capsules can be added to mixture to prolong the life of oil up to one year.

Herbal teas (Infusion)

Herbal tea mixtures can be placed in a tea ball if loose or made into tea bags by using tea bags that seal with an iron.

Decoction

Herb is placed in glass or enamel saucepan with cold water and slowly brought to a boil, reduce heat and simmer for 10 minutes and steep with lid on for 3 minutes. This method is used for barks such as liquorice and will keep up to three days refrigerated.

Tincture

Put 4 ounces powdered herb or 8 ounces fresh chopped herb in a container with tightly fitted lid add 1 pint alcohol, 60% proof brandy or vodka. Stand the mixture in a warm place and shake it twice daily for 2 weeks. Strain through cheesecloth, squeezing out liquid and store in a well sealed dark glass jar.

Ointments and creams

Prepare and strain a strong decoction or infusion of the herb and add to a pure cold-pressed vegetable oil, boil till liquid has evaporated. To stiffen as a cream, stir in melted beeswax *(Cera alba)* 1 ounce good for 1 1/4 cups of oil. Add a drop of tincture of Benzoin or Myrrh or a Vitamin E capsule to extend its life. Coconut *(Cocos nucifera)* or Cocoa Butter *(Theobroma cacoa)* or an aloe vera gel *(Aloe barbadensis)* are often added for a creamier more moisturizing consistency.

Hot and Cold Compresses

For a hot compress soak a clean linen or cotton cloth in a hot decoction or infusion and apply it to the affected part as hot as can be tolerated. Cover compress with plastic wrap and put a hot water bottle on it to maintain the heat. To prepare a cold compress use same method, but allow to cool before applying.

Poultice

In a poultice plant parts are used rather than liquid extraction. Mash or crush fresh plant parts and either heat in a pot over boiling water or mix with a small amount of boiling water. Apply pulp directly to the skin and hold in place with a gauze bandage. If using a dried herb, first powder it and make a paste with a little boiling water, if a skin irritant, apply between two layers of cloth. Poultices are used to stimulate circulation, soothe aches and pains or draw impurities out through the skin.

8 HERBAL TEAS

Adaptogen Teas

Blood Builder Tea

1 tsp Rose Hips-crushed

1 Tsp Butcher's Broom

1 Tsp Yellow Dock

Bring 3 1/2 cups of water to a boil. Remove water from heat and add herbs. Place a tight lid on the pot. Let the mixture steep for five to ten minutes. Drink one cup three times daily. Yields three cups.

Blossoms of Health Tea

Beautiful to look at, nectar to taste and good for you. A popular tea. Spirited, uplifting and energizing.

1 part Ginkgo leaves

1 part Red clover tops

1 part Nettle leaves

1 part Meadowsweet leaves

1 part Calendula

2 parts Chamomile

2 parts Lavender flowers

1 part Gotu Kola leaves

a pinch of stevia.

Place all herbs in a tea ball or bag, put in your nicest or most favorite cup or mug, and cover with boiling water. Steep for 10 minutes. Remove tea ball or bag, and add sugar, honey, sweetener, milk, cream or whatever, to taste.

Echinacea & Roots Tea

A tasty way to help strengthen and support your natural resistance. A very popular tea.

1 part Echinacea Purpurea root

1 part Pau D'arco

1 part Dandelion root (raw and roasted)

1 part Sarsaparilla bark

1 part Cinnamon barks

1 part Ginger root

1 part Burdock roots

1 part Sassafras bark

a pinch of stevia

Place all herbs in a tea ball or bag, put in your nicest or most favorite cup or mug, and cover with boiling water. Steep for 10 minutes. Remove tea ball or bag, and add sugar, honey, sweetener, milk, cream or whatever, to taste.

Tea For Health

1 tablespoon China black tea

2 teaspoon Fennel

1 teaspoon Mint

2 teaspoon Rose hips

1 teaspoon Elder flower

2 teaspoon Hops

1 teaspoon Mullein

Constipation Tea

1/2 teaspoon Cascara sagrada

1 teaspoon Chamomile

Take in one dose before bedtime. One coffee cup full should do it.

Detox Tea

1 Teaspoon Pau D'Arco (Taheebo)

1 Teaspoon Cascara sagrada

1 Teaspoon Echinacea

Bring 1 1/2 cups water to a boil. Place herbs into the water, cover tightly and let steep for five minutes. 1 cup two times a day should help. If bowels are loose, dilute combination in 2 to 2 1/2 cups water.

Allergies

Allergy Season Blend

Cool minty, citrus flavour to assist you with the discomfort associated with allergy season.

1 part Nettle

1 part Peppermint

1 part Spearmint

1 part Yerba santa

1 part Eyebright

1 part Lemongrass leaves

1 part Calendula

1 part Red clover

1 part Lavender flowers

1 part Fennel seeds

a pinch of stevia

Place all herbs in a tea ball or bag, put in your nicest or most favorite cup or mug, and cover with boiling water. Steep for 10 minutes. Remove tea ball or bag, and add sugar, honey, sweetener, milk, cream or whatever, to taste.

During cold or sinus season Tea

1 small handful (about 1/4 cup) dried Thyme

1 small handful (about 1/4 cup) dried Feverfew flowers

1 large handful (about 3/4 cup) dried Peppermint leaves

1 Tablespoon dried and rubbed or crushed Sage

Bladder Infections

Bladder Infections Tea

1 ½ oz dried Goldenrod

1/4 oz Juniper Berries*

3/4 oz chopped Dandelion root

3/4 oz chopped Rose Hips

Pour 1 cup boiling water over 2 tsp of mixture. Steep 10 minutes & strain. *can become toxic, so only drink 2 cups of this mixture daily for no more than 3 days*

Bad Chest Teas

Bronchial Congestion Tea

1 ½ oz Aniseed

1 oz Calendula flowers

3/4 oz Marshmallow root

1/3 oz Licorice root

Crush aniseeds and add to herbs. Pour 1 cup boiling water over 1 tsp mixture; cover & steep 10 minutes.

Colds and Flu Tea

1 oz Blackberry leaves

1 oz Elder flowers

1 oz Linden flowers

1 oz Peppermint leaves

Pour 1 cup boiling water over 2 tbls. mixture. Cover & steep 10 minutes; strain.

Colds and Hoarseness Tea

2 oz Malva flowers

1 ½ oz Mullein flowers

Use 2 Tbls of mixture per 1 cup hot water. Steep 10 minutes; strain. Drink only 2 - 3 cups per day for just a few days.

Stop that Cough Tea

1 tablespoon Slippery Elm

1 tablespoon Mullein

1 tablespoon Catnip

1 tablespoon Licorice root bark

Boil the bark first in two cups worth of water for 10 minutes. Place the rest of the herbs in a coffee filter and place the filter in a strainer. Strain the Licorice tea through the strainer into a mug and drink.

Honey and lemon can be added.

Winter Tea

Boneset

Echinacea

Peppermint

Just use equal parts of each, or pre-made tea bags...3 bags, 1 of Boneset,1 of Echinacea, and 1 of Peppermint.

The Echinacea works as an immune system builder, the boneset is great for congestion, aches and fever (the classic flu symptoms), and the Peppermint aids with any stomach complaints due to drainage from the sinuses, and just works as a great overall "feel-good".

Coughing Fits Tea

1 1/3 oz. St. John's Wort
2/3 oz. Thyme
2/3 oz. Linden Flowers

Use 1 tsp. of the herb mixture per cup of boiling water to soothe irritations of the upper respiratory tract that cause coughing. Steep for 5-10 min., strain, sweeten if necessary. This tea has proved helpful with bronchitis and whooping cough.

Fever Reducer Tea

2 tsp dried Catnip

1 tsp dry Vervain

Pour 2 cups boiling water over herbs. Steep 10 minutes & strain.

Flu-away

2 medium cloves of freshly crushed Garlic

1 cup of very warm water

1 teaspoon of honey

1 teaspoon of lemon juice

Stir and drink.

Forests Tea (formerly Lung Blend)

1 part Echinacea purpurea

1 part Elecampane

1 part Ginger

1 part each Pleurisy & Licorice roots

1 part White oak bark

1 part Cinnamon bark

1 part each Orange peel and Fennel seeds

Place all herbs in a tea ball or bag, put in your nicest or most favorite cup or mug, and cover with boiling water. Steep for 10 minutes. Remove tea ball or bag, and add sugar, honey, sweetener, milk, cream or whatever, to taste.

Sore throat Tea

Licorice root

Slippery Elm

Peppermint

The Common Cold

1 1/2 tablespoons of Licorice root already brewed in a pot enough for two cups.

Elderberry tea bag

Chamomile

Steep the tea bag in the Licorice Root infusion and add in the Chamomile. This can be done in the coffee maker, but the Licorice brew must be cool enough to be cycled through the machine.

Calming Teas

Calming Tea 1

1 oz Lemon balm

1 oz Chamomile flowers

½ oz St John's Wort

Steep 2 tbs of mixture in 1 cup boiled water. Cover 10 minutes; strain.

Calming Tea 2

1 Part Sage

1 Part Thyme

1 Part Marjoram

1 Part Chamomile

Blend ingredients in a tea ball and put in a mug of hot water

End of Your Rope Tea

1 Tablespoon Chamomile

1 Tablespoon Peppermint

Put in a tea ball and steep in boiling hot water for five minutes.

Less Stress Tea

Relieves stress, relaxes low back and neck areas.

1 part Chamomile

1 part Mint

1 part Calendula flowers

Place all herbs in a tea ball or bag, put in your nicest or most favorite cup or mug, and cover with boiling water. Steep for 10 minutes. Remove tea ball or bag, and add sugar, honey, sweetener, milk, cream or whatever, to taste.

Mellow Mood Tea

This tea is made with the most palatable of the calming herbs. Blended together, they'll defuse stress and anxiety and promote sound sleep.

1 teaspoon Chamomile flowers

1 teaspoon Lavender spikes

1 teaspoon Kava leaves

1 teaspoon Lemon Balm leaves

1 teaspoon Marjoram

1 spray Valerian flowers

1 quart water

In a large saucepan, steep the Chamomile, Lavender, Kava, Lemon balm, Marjoram, and Valerian to taste in the freshly boiled water. Strain out the plant material. Drink the tea hot or cool as often as needed, refrigerating any left over for later use. **CAUTION: Chamomile is in the rag weed family.**

My Nerves Are Shot Tea!

Uses: Sleeplessness and Insomnia

Job-related stress, Panic attacks

Ingredients:

2 parts Chamomile

1 part Jasmine

1 part Hops

1 part Lavender

1 part Yerba Santa

1 part Gota Kola

1 part St. John's Wort

Preparation:

Place all herbs in a tea ball or bag, put in your nicest or most favorite cup or mug, and cover with boiling water. Steep for 10 minutes. Remove tea ball or bag, and add sugar, honey, sweetener, milk, cream or whatever, to taste.

Pleasant Dreams

1 cup Mugwort

1/2 cup Rose petals

1/2 cup Chamomile

1/3 cup Lavender flowers

1/3 cup Catnip

2 tbsp Mint

Quiet Child Tea

Good for anytime of the day or right before bedtime.

1 part Raspberry leaves

1 part Catnip

1 part each Spearmint & Skullcap leaves

1 part Calendula flowers

a pinch of stevia

Place all herbs in a tea ball or bag, put in your nicest or most favorite cup or mug, and cover with boiling water. Steep for 10 minutes. Remove tea ball or bag, and add sugar, honey, sweetener, milk, cream or whatever, to taste.

Quiet Time Tea

1 part Oregano

2 parts Chamomile

1 part Lemon Balm

1 part Lemon Thyme

Place all herbs in a tea ball or bag, put in your nicest or most favorite cup or mug, and cover with boiling water. Steep for 10 minutes. Remove tea ball or bag, and add sugar, honey, sweetener, milk, cream or whatever, to taste.

Stress-Reducing Rest

1/2 cup Sweet Hops

1/2 cup Mugwort

1/8 cup Sweet Marjoram

All the following recipes have the same measurements. Unless otherwise stated, they were brewed in a coffee maker or tea brewer.

Measurements: 1 tablespoon of each type of herb 1 tablespoon of honey to sweeten the tea

Rejuvenation Tea

Etheric cleanser of old, stale thoughts and patterns of behavior for new beginnings and awakening.

1 part Rose hips

1 part Calendula flowers

1 part Gallum (cleavers) flowers

1 part Borage flowers

1 part Nettles leaves

Place all herbs in a tea ball or bag, put in your nicest or most favorite cup or mug, and cover with boiling water. Steep for 10 minutes. Remove tea ball or bag, and add sugar, honey, sweetener, milk, cream or whatever, to taste.

Relaxation Tea

2 parts Chamomile

1 part Lemon Balm

1 part Lemon peel

1 part Thyme

Place all herbs in a tea ball or bag, put in your nicest or most favorite cup or mug, and cover with boiling water. Steep for 10 minutes. Remove tea ball or bag, and add sugar, honey, sweetener, milk, cream or whatever, to taste.

Sleep Tea Recipe

2 tbls. Hops

1 tsp. Lavender

1 tsp. Rosemary

1 tsp. Thyme

1 tsp. Mugwort

1 tsp. Sage

1 Pinch of Valerian Root

Take a teaspoon of the mixture and pour into 1 cup of hot water. Let sit for 3 minutes then strain. Store the unused portion.

Soothing Tea

1 part Mint

1 part Hyssop

1 part Oregano

1 part Parsley

1 part Lemon balm

Place all herbs in a tea ball or bag, put in your nicest or most favorite cup or mug, and cover with boiling water. Steep for 10 minutes. Remove tea ball or bag, and add sugar, honey, sweetener, milk, cream or whatever, to taste.

Spiced Relief

1 teaspoon Anise seeds, crushed or ground

2-3 Cinnamon sticks

1 inch of Ginger, sliced

1-2 teaspoons dried loose Echinacea

Combine spices and Echinacea in a pot with three cups of water. Bring to a boil and then simmer for 15-20 minutes to make a decoction. Strain into a mug and add honey to taste. This is a multifunction tea. Anise acts as an expectorant, ginger soothes the cough, and cinnamon has anti-bacterial properties.

Super Relaxer Tea

1 part (1 teaspoon) Valerian root (dried)

1 part (1 teaspoon) Chamomile flowers (dried)

In a Teapot pour in 2 mug full of hot water (not boiling) steep for 5 mins. Strain or remove tea bags. Add honey if desired. This is great at night before bed.

Tranquility Tea

Mix:

2 parts Red Clover blossoms

2 parts Rose Hips

1 part German Chamomile flowers

1 part Peppermint leaves

Baby Sleep Tea

1 tsp Hops

1 tsp Chamomile

Place 4 cups of water into a glass or porcelain pot and bring to a boil. Take the pot off the heat and add the herbs. Put a tight lid on the pot and let it steep for five minutes. Strain out herbs. Place in four ounce glass bottle after it is cool enough for baby and let them drink it.

Depression Teas

Blues Tea

1 part Nettle leaves,

1 part St John's Wort tops

2 parts Spearmint

1 part Damiana leaves

1 part Kava kava root

a tiny pinch of stevia to taste

Place all herbs in a tea ball or bag, put in your nicest or most favorite cup or mug, and cover with boiling water. Steep for 10 minutes. Remove tea ball or bag, and add sugar, honey, sweetener, milk, cream or whatever, to taste.

Depression Tamer Tea

1 tsp St John's Wort

1 tsp Gingko Biloba

Place 1 cup of water into a glass or porcelain pot and bring to a boil.

Take the pot of the heat and add the herbals. Put a tight lid on the pot and let it steep for five minutes. Strain out herbals. Place in a cup and sweeten with honey of desired.

Headache, Bad Tummy

Happy Tummy Tea

Put a smile on your face with this soothing and yummy tea.

1 part Catnip

1 part Spearmint & Lemongrass leaves

1 part Calendula flowers

1 part Skullcap

1 part Rosemary & Sage leaves

1 part Fennel seeds

Place all herbs in a tea ball or bag, put in your nicest or most favorite cup or mug, and cover with boiling water. Steep for 10 minutes. Remove tea ball or bag, and add sugar, honey, sweetener, milk, cream or whatever, to taste.

Pinkeye tea recipe

Fill a tea ball with equal parts chamomile (antiseptic), borage (alleviated inflammation and redness), eyebright (excellent for conjunctivitis any other eye complaints) and elderflowers (beneficial for tired eyes). Pour on 2 1/2 cups boiling hot (fresh from the kettle) water allow to steep until cooled. Add 5 drops witch hazel extract (coolant and antiseptic) and stir.

Wash eye (outside) gently with infusion and put one drop of infusion in eye as needed or desired. Also can be used by soaking a cloth in the infusion and putting over the eye until you eye feels better. If your using this for a child leave out the witch hazel. This is good for anything where your eyes are painful inflamed and red.

Headache Tea

Lavender

Chamomile

Rosemary

Mint

Put a pinch of each herb in a coffee filter and place in your coffee maker. Wait a half hour before drinking this mix, this should make you tired so you can sleep your headache away.

Patti's Pain Killer Tea

The herbs you can choose from are as follows:

Lady´s Mantle (herb)

Raspberry Leaf (herb)

Yarrow (herb)

Chaste Tree Berry

Fennel Seed (for the stomach)

Peppermint (for the stomach)

Valerian (for the stomach)

Use (1) part each (choose a total of five including one for the stomach) and steep like a tea.

Healing Ginger tea

2 cups of water

4 tablespoons freshly grated ginger root

Place in pan with a lid on, bring to a boil, turn off the heat and let sit for two hours. Re-heat the tea, strain the herb from the tea and drink.

Nervous Stomach Tea

2 tsp Angelica root

2 tsp Lemon Balm leaves

½ tsp Fennel seed

Bring Angelica root to a simmer in 4 cups water. Turn off heat, add lemon balm & lemon; steep 10 minutes & strain.

Nervous Tension Tea

1 1/3 oz. St. John's Wort

1 oz. Lemon Balm Leaves

1 oz. Valerian

Use 1 tsp of the herb mixture per cup of boiling water. Steep for 10 min., strain, sweeten if necessary. Drink a cup before going to bed each night for several weeks to calm nerves, lifts Depression, and help you fall asleep more easily.

Heartburn Tea

1 tablespoon Chamomile

1 table spoon Peppermint

2 pods Star Anise

Boil pods for 5 minutes and steep the chamomile and peppermint in the Anise tea. Drink one cup every hour for two hours before bedtime.

Memory Zest Blend

A mentally refreshing beverage, to help give you feelings of clarity and precision.

1 part Ginkgo

1 part Gotu Kola and Peppermint leaves

1 part Red Clover tops

1 part Rosemary leaves

1 part Ginger root

a pinch of stevia.

Place all herbs in a tea ball or bag, put in your nicest or most favorite cup or mug, and cover with boiling water. Steep for 10 minutes.

Remove tea ball or bag, and add sugar, honey, sweetener, milk, cream or whatever, to taste.

Migraine Tea

1 2/3 oz dried St. John's Wort

1 oz Valerian

1 oz Linden flowers

1/4 oz Juniper berries

Use 1 tsp of mixture per 1 cup boiling water. Steep 10 minutes & strain.

Aches and Pains Tea

1 Tablespoon White Willow Bark

1 Tablespoon Catnip

Put in a tea ball and steep in boiling hot water for five minutes. Drink as hot as you can stand it, then lie down for a nap.

Love Teas

Aphrodite Blend Tea

A sensuous, aromatic blend with just the right tint of zest for your palate, and sure to kindle flames! A delicate, but dashing combination makes this one of your most enjoyable cups of tea.

1 part Damiana leaves

1 part Rose petals

1 part Peppermint leaves

1 part Muira Puama

1 part Gingko leaves

1 part Orange peel

1 part Cinnamon bark chips

pinch of stevia.

Place all herbs in a tea ball or bag, put in your nicest or most favorite cup or mug, and cover with boiling water. Steep for 10 minutes. Remove tea ball or bag, and add sugar, honey, sweetener, milk.

Happy Man Tea Blend

1 part Siberian ginseng

1 part Dandelion root

1 part Nettle

1 part each Marshmallow & Burdock roots

1 part each Hawthorn & Saw Palmetto berries

1 part Fennel seeds

1 part Wild Oats

a pinch of stevia

Place all herbs in a tea ball or bag, put in your nicest or most favorite cup or mug, and cover with boiling water. Steep for 10 minutes. Remove tea ball or bag, and add sugar, honey, sweetener, milk, cream

or whatever, to taste. Climb into bed and enjoy!

Menstrual Cramps

Dual Purpose Tea

Do not drink more than 2 cups a day.

2 teaspoons dried German Chamomile flowers

1 cup boiling water

Steep the flowers in the boiling water, covered, for 15 minutes. Strain, then slowly sip the infusion to relieve nausea, stomach upset, and lessen menstrual cramps.

Cramp Tea

1 teaspoon Cramp Bark

1 teaspoon Red Raspberry Leaves

1 teaspoon Dong Quai

Take this tea in coffee cup full glasses. This makes enough for two cups. The tea is only good for six hours.

Tea for menstrual problems, fertility and childbirth

3 tablespoons Sassafras bark

2 tablespoons Dandelion root

1 tablespoon Ginger root

½ tablespoon Cinnamon

1 tablespoon Licorice root

½ tablespoon Orange peel

1 tablespoon Pau d'arco

¼ tablespoon Dong Quai root

1 tablespoon Chasteberry

1 tablespoon Wild Yam

Place all herbs in a tea ball or bag, put in your nicest or most favorite cup or mug, and cover with boiling water. Steep for 10 minutes. Remove tea ball or bag, and add sugar, honey, sweetener, milk.

Moon Ease Tea

For that time of the month.

2 parts Crampbark

1 part Chaste tree berries

1 part each Spearmint & Skullcap leaves

1 part Marshmallow root

1 part Passionflower herb

1 part Ginger root

Procedure: Place all herbs in a tea ball or bag, put in your nicest or most favorite cup or mug, and cover with boiling water. Steep for 10 minutes. Remove tea ball or bag, and add sugar, honey, sweetener, milk, cream or whatever, to taste.

Menopause Tea

Crone Root Tea

For menopause and beginning a new cycle of life.

2 tablespoons Wild yam

2 tablespoons Licorice

3 tablespoons Sarsaparilla

1 tablespoon Chaste berry

1 tablespoon Ginger

1 tablespoon False Unicorn root

2 tablespoons Sage

1 tablespoon Cinnamon

½ tablespoon Black Cohash

Place all herbs in a tea ball or bag, put in your nicest or most favorite cup or mug, and cover with boiling water. Steep for 10 minutes.

Remove tea ball or bag, and add sugar, honey, sweetener, milk, cream or whatever, to taste.

Flashes Blend Tea

Brew up a pot and sip when needed.

1 part Sage

1 part Motherwort

1 part Dandelion

1 part Chickweed & Violet leaves

1 part each Elder flowers & Oatstraw

Place all herbs in a tea ball or bag, put in your nicest or most favorite cup or mug, and cover with boiling water. Steep for 10 minutes. Remove tea ball or bag, and add sugar, honey, sweetener, milk, cream or whatever, to taste.

Breast Health Tea

2 parts Calendula

2 parts Red Clover

1 part Cleavers

1 part Lady's Mantle

Spearmint or Peppermint (optional; for flavor)

Prepare as an infusion, using 1 ounce of herbs per quart of water, and letting steep overnight. Drink 3 to 4 cups daily.

Wise Woman Tea

A wonderful menopause tea. Gently calms, cools and balances.

1 part Motherwort

1 part Sage

1 part Nettle leaves

1 part each Lemon balm & Mugwort leaves

1 part Chaste tree berries

1 part Horsetail

Place all herbs in a tea ball or bag, put in your nicest or most favorite cup or mug, and cover with boiling water. Steep for 10 minutes. Remove tea ball or bag, and add sugar, honey, sweetener, milk, cream or whatever, to taste.

Sleep Tea

Dream Tea

2 parts Rose

1 part Mugwort

1 part Peppermint

1 part Jasmine

1/2 part Cinnamon

Drink to cause dreams.

Combine all ingredients thoroughly; fill tea diffuser with 1 tsp. per cup of boiling water.

Evening Repose Tea

When the sun sets over the hill and the new moon dips her silver softness, savour the tranquility in our evening repose blend. It's a perfect toast to the rising moon. A robust flavour of flowers and mint.

1 part Roses

1 part Lavender flowers

1 part Lemon verbena leaves

1 part Chamomile flowers

1 part each Peppermint & Spearmint leaves

1 part Blue Malva flowers

pinch of stevia

Place all herbs in a tea ball or bag, put in your nicest or most favorite cup or mug, and cover with boiling water. Steep for 10 minutes. Remove tea ball or bag, and add sugar, honey, sweetener, milk, cream or whatever, to taste.

Insomnia Tea

1 ½ oz dried Vervain leaves

1 oz Chamomile

½ oz Spearmint

Mix all and add to 1 cup boiling water. Steep 8 minutes; strain.

9 CHAPTER NAME

Prepare dye bath by soaking the herb in water overnight and then boiling until the colour has been extracted. Strain and use 18 litres of dye bath to a pound dry weight of material. For wool, cotton or linen, simmer in the dye bath for as long as necessary to achieve desired dolour. For silk keep the temperature below 71 degrees Celsius.

To mordant clean material is simmered (wool) boiled (cotton, linen) soaker in hot water (silk) in which the chemical has been dissolved

Rinse a number of times, each one a little cooler than the last, until the rinse water remains clear.

Plant	Part Used	Color	Material	Mordant
Alder	Bark	Grey/ Brown	Wool	Ferrous Sulphate
Alder	Bark	Brown/ Yellow	Cotton	Alum
Alder	Leaves	Green Yellow	Wool	Alum
Alder Buck Thorn	Bark	Bronze	Wool	

Plant	Part Used	Color	Material	Mordant
Alkanet	Root	Red	Wool	
Almond	Leaves	Yellow	Wool	Alum
Cranberry	Stems/Leaves	Yellow/ Red	Wool Linen	Alum
Apple Tree	Bark	Yellow	Wool	
Barberry	Leaves	Black	Wool	Ferrous Sulphate
Blackberry	Leaves	Black	Wool	Ferrous Sulphate
Blackthorn	Bark	Red/ Brown/ Black	Wool	Ferrous Sulphate
Bloodroot	Root	Red/ Orange Yellow	Wool	Alum
Bracken	Roots, Young Shoots	Yellow Yellow Green/Grey	Wool/Silk Silk	Chrome Alum Ferrous Sulphate
Coltsfoot	Herb	Yellow/ Green	Wool Wool	Alum Ferrous Sulphate
Cornflower	Flowers	Blue	Wool	
Dandelion	Root	Magenta	Wool	
Dog's Mercy	Herb	Green Yellow/Blue	Wool	
Dyer's Bed-Straw	Roots	Red	Wool	
Dyer's Broom	Flowering Top Tops	Yellow Green	Wool	Alum dye Over Indigo
Elder	Fruit	Violet Lilac	Wool	Alum Alum/Salt
Goldenrod	Flowers	Yellow	Wool	Alum/Chrome
Heather	Young Flowers Plant Top After Flower	Green Yellow	Wool	Alum None Alum
Iceland Moss	Lichen	Brown	Wool	
Juniper	Berries	Brown	Wool	
Lady's Mantel	Green parts	Green	Wool	
Larch	Needles	Brown	Wool	
Larkspur	Flowers	Green	Wool	Alum
Madder	Roots	Laquer Red	Wool	Alum
Madder	Roots	Garnet	Wool	Chrome

Plant	Part Used	Color	Material	Mordant
Marigold	Petals	Yellow	Wool/Silk	Alum
Meadow-	Tops	Green	Wool	Alum
Sweet	Roots	Yellow	Wool	None
		Black		
Nettle	Herb	Green	Wool	Alum
Onion	Outside	Burnt	Wool	Alum
	Skin	Orange	Wool	Chrome
		Brass		
		Green	Wool	Ferrous S.
Oak	Bark	Black	Wool	Ferrous S.
Ragwort	Herb	Yellow	Wool	Alum
Rowan	Bark	Grey	Wool	
St. John's Wort	Tops	Yellow	Wool	Alum
Sorrel	Leaves	Green	Wool	
		Yellow		
Tansy	Leaves	Yellow	Wool	
		Green		
Tea	Leaves	Rose-tan	Wool	
Walnut	Green	Dark	Wool	Alum
	Hulls of nuts	Brown		
Wild Crab Apple	Bark	Yellow	Wool	
Yellow Dock	Roots	Black	Wool	Chrome

Further Herbal Dye Resources

http://www.georgeweil.co.uk/
http://www.handmadepresents.co.uk/
http://www.knitting-and-crochet-guild.org.uk/
http://www.theloomexchange.co.uk/
http://www.naturaldyes.org/
http://www.onlineguildwsd.org.uk/
http://wildcolours.co.uk/
http://www.wsd.org.uk/links.htm

10 MAKING POTPOURRI & INCENSE

Potpourri is a beautiful use of herbs that is visually as well as aromatically appealing. Muslin bags can be made that contain hops, lavender, plantain and corn flour for sleeping and sweet violet bags for a bad chest. Lavender and rose bags have been traditionally used to freshen chest of drawers and cedar wood chips to prevent moths.

Country Garden Potpourri

2 cups Rose petals
1 cup Rosebuds
2 cups Lavender
1 cup mock Orange flowers
1 cup scented Pelargonium leaves
1 cup pinks
1 cup Bee balm leaves
1 cup Larkspur flowers ¼ cup daisies
8 Love-in-a-mist sweet capsules or hop flowers
8 Helichrysum flowers
5 tbsp Orris root.

Elizabethan Mixture
2 cups Lemon Verbena
2 cups Lavender flowers
1 cup Bearberry leaves
1 cup Sweet myrtle leaves
1 cup Delphiniums
½ cup Violets
½ cup Blue mallow flowers

½ cup crushed Roseroot
1 oz Rosewood
1 tbsp Orris root
1 tbsp gum Benzoin

Fly-away potpourri

2 cups Lavender flowers
1 cup Rosemary
1 cup Southernwood
1/2 cup Spearmint
½ cup Santolina
¼ cup Pennyroyal
¼ cup Tansy
¼ cup Cedarwood chips
10 yellow tulips
3 Tbsp Orris root

Marigold, Lemon and Mint Mix

500 ml (1 pint) mixed Marigold and Chamomile flowers
500 ml (1 pint) mixed Lemon balm and mint
50 g (2 oz) Lavender
25 g (1 oz) Rosemary
25 g (1 oz) Orris root powder
½ Cinnamon stick
1 strip Lemon peel
½ teaspoon whole Cloves
½ teaspoon grated Nutmeg
3 drops Geranium oil
2 drops Lemon oil
1 drop Peppermint oil
Flowers to decorate (Parsley, Anaphalis and Blue Larkspur)

Pomanders Balls

2 medium-sized thin-skinned Oranges
Whole Cloves
Orris root powder
Cinnamon powder
Allspice powder
Nutmeg powder

Mix the powders together. Stick the cloves into the oranges. Roll in the powder. Place in a bowl beside heat.

Pretty Victorian Potpourri

5oo ml (1 pint) mixed pink, mauve or cream, scented material from the following: Rose buds, Violet, pink, Chamomile flowers and Heliotrope
500 ml (1 pint) mixed Thyme, Rosemary, Myrtle, sweet Cicely leaves and Bergamot
25 g (i oz) Lavender
25 g (i oz Orris root powder
25 g (1 oz) fine-ground gum Benzoin
½ Cinnamon stick
½ tsp whole Cloves
½ tsp ground Allspice
2 drops Rose oil
2 drops Lavender oil
2 drops Lemon oil
Pink and mauve flowers to decorate

Rose & Mint Potpourri

1 lb Rose petals
½ tsp Cinnamon
½ tsp crushed Cloves
½ tsp Nutmeg
1 tsp Mint
2 tsp Devil's claw
3 drops Rose essential oil
Combine dried flowers and leaves in a large bowl. Add spices. Drop oil onto rose petals and combine all ingredients thoroughly. Store in a sealed container for at least one month before using. Shake well before use.

Soothing Potpourris

2 cups Lemon Verbena
2 cups Rose petals
1 cup Lavender flowers
1 cup Calendula petals
1 cup Meadowsweet florets
1 cup Chamomile flowers

1 oz Angelica root
4 tbsp Orris root

Wedding Potpourri

1 litre (1 quart) mixed white and pink Rose petals, Orange blossom, Myrtle flowers, White Hydrangea flowers, pink Rose buds, and any other flowers from the bridal bouquet.

50 g (2 oz) mixed Myrtle leaves, Basil, Rose leaves, and Marjoram
25 g (1 oz Rosemary
25 g (1 oz) fine-ground gum Benzoin
25 g (1 oz) Orris root powder
1 crushed Cardamom
1 teaspoon crushed Cassia
3 drops Rose oil
2 drops Lavender oil
1 drop Patchouli oil
Silver-sprayed flowers to decorate

Incense

These are incense you can make yourself. Put on a fire safe base, with a charcoal disk, light disk and put incense over it to burn.

Psychic Protection Incense

1 part Broom
½ part Agrimony
½ part Basil
½ part Oregano

Samhain Incense

2 parts Cinnamon
1 part Ground Cloves
1 part Dragon's Blood resin
1 part Hyssop
1 part Patchouli
2 parts Rosemary
1 part Sage
A dash of sea salt

Sun Incense

3 parts Frankincense
2 parts Myrrh
1 part Balm of Gilead
½ part bay leaves
½ part Calendula petals
2 drops Musk Oil and 2 drops Olive Oil

Summer of Love Incense

2 parts Catnip
2 parts Chamomile blossoms
1 part Lavender blossoms
1 part Patchouli
1/2 part Sweet Annie

Further Resources

http://www.bushcraft-magazine.co.uk/

http://www.emedicinal.com/

http://www.healthmonthly.co.uk

http://www.herbalgram.org/

http://www.herbs.org/

http://www.herbsociety.org.uk/

http://www.naturalark.com/

http://www.pfaf.org/index.php

http://www.rbgkew.org.uk/

http://www.yourhealthfoodstore.co.uk

Herbal Suppliers

The Alchemists Apothecary

http://stores.shop.ebay.co.uk/The-Alchemists-Apothecary

http://www.aromantic.co.uk/

www.baldwins.co.uk

www.herbmoonhollow.com

U.S.A.

http://www.blessedherbs.com/

http://www.brambleberry.com/

http://www.bulkapothecary.com/

INDEX

ABOUT THE AUTHOR

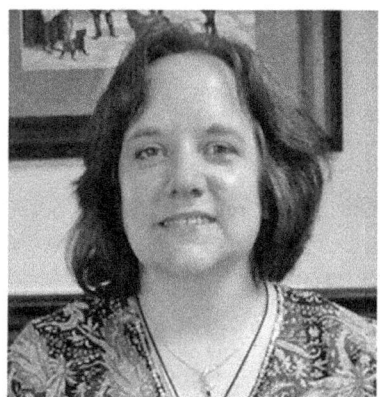

Cara E. Moore is a writer, poet and playwright who writes for Newspapers, Magazines and Internet sites, and whose play, The Healing won an honorable mention in the 1996 Writer's Digest Playwright Competition. She is the author of a collection of poetry <u>Horizon's Place And Time Meet</u>. She is also a Crystal Healing and Herbalism Practitioner and a Hatha Yoga Teacher, training at the British School of Yoga. She runs courses in Herbalism accredited by the World Metaphysical Association and has formulated a range of health and beauty products Crystal Essence ® available from Crystal Arts And Health.